FEED YOUR KIDS RIGHT

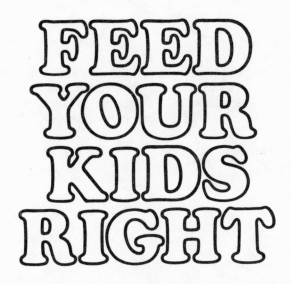

FEED YOUR KIDS RIGHT

DR. SMITH'S PROGRAM FOR YOUR CHILD'S TOTAL HEALTH

LENDON SMITH, M.D.

McGraw-Hill Book Company

New York   St. Louis   San Francisco
Düsseldorf   Mexico   Toronto

This book is not intended to replace the services
of a physician. Any application of the
recommendations set forth in the following pages
is at the reader's discretion and sole risk.

1 2 3 4 5 6 7 8 9 0 FGRFGR 7 9 8 3 2 1 0 9

LIBRARY OF CONGRESS CATALOGING IN PUBLICATION DATA
Smith, Lendon H,
   Feed your kids right.
   Includes index.
   1. Children—Nutrition.   2. Children—Diseases—
Nutritional aspects.   I. Title.
RJ206.S62   613.2   78-23733
ISBN 0-07-058496-6

Book design by Marsha Picker

To my wife, Juliet Smith,
who has fed my body and my brain
for the last thirty years

Preface

When I began pediatric practice almost three decades ago, I was unaware of the value of a nutritional approach to treating children's diseases and behaviors. As medical students we had been taught that Americans were the best-fed people on earth and that only quacks used nutrition in the treatment of disease.

Today, after so many years of observing and treating children, I am convinced that the best overall approach for our kids is the provision—beginning even before the mother's pregnancy—of emotional and physical nutrients.

Child rearing should be fun; if it isn't fun, it won't work. Parents should be able to laugh more than they cry, but what I see in many cases are vicious cycles of ill health that get started needlessly, largely through parents' ignorance of preventive health approaches. Mothers and fathers have been worrying about the wrong things and failing to do what they should about some terribly important symptoms and behaviors.

Most young mothers are afraid to take a strong stand on sound family nutrition. Many are afraid that their children will not love them if they do not provide sweet foods. Many feel they will poison their children if they give them extra vitamins and minerals but at the same time casually shovel antibiotics, antihistamines, and tranquilizers into them simply because a doctor says it is okay to do so.

The role of the medical practitioner has been to treat symptoms with the medicines at his disposal. It is time to add the preventive approach to the traditional curative approach. The two are not mutually exclusive. The medical practitioner should be able to plot the individual needs of each of his patients by taking the medical history (family diseases, personality traits, susceptibility to stress and infection, birth history, pregnancy problems), giving a physical examination (including blood pressure, heart rate, body size and shape, and condition of skin, nails, and teeth), and ordering appropriate blood, urine, and hair studies.

We are all different biochemically and have different nutritional needs. What works for me may not work for you. I alone can perceive all my stresses and mental and physical symptoms. I alone must plan my health. If 500 mg of vitamin C a day prevents me from having a nosebleed, am I cheating if I take it?

I hope the holistic health professionals as well as my prescription-writing colleagues will forgive my effrontery in writing this book. It represents a new beginning for me, as I hope it will for the people who read it. Its purpose is to chart the path to good health with less medicine. Give it a try. It's safe. It's sound. Then, at the next checkup for your child, if you report fewer allergies and infections, better sleep and behavior, and the doctor says your child is in great shape, you will be able to smile. You will know why.

I am indebted to and have been encouraged by the following people who feel that this book is a valid approach to better physical and mental health.

Mr. Ray Gilman, pharmacist, has been most helpful in providing many of the biochemical insights. He is also aware of the disappointments patients suffer when provided with therapy that treats only the symptoms.

Mrs. Linda Davis of Streamwood, Illinois, has seen the bad effects of poor nutrition in her classes. She has organized a supportive group of concerned parents (Sugarholics United to Guard Against Relapse) to help encourage the initial motivation.

Mr. Richard Meshbesher of Minneapolis, president of the Middle Atlantic Health Organization, feels my concern for health coincides with his. He wanted this book titled *Doctor Smith Says It's OK*.

Mr. John O'Farrell Gleason of Portland has reinforced my work and is developing a system of better nutrition.

My patients were willing to follow these ideas and of course were rewarded with better health.

My wife has been the most supportive of all. She thinks the book could have been shortened and summarized into two words: *common sense*.

L. S.

Contents

The 1
Five Levels
of Health

The theory on which this book is based is that optimal nutrition will maintain a person in health that is optimal for his or her particular genetic endowment. We could all be healthier than we are, and the failure to achieve an elevated plateau is directly proportional to the degree and significance of our various nutritional deficiencies. I am proposing here that the right food and appropriate nutritional supplements can maintain and improve health and forestall the development of illness.

Picture a somewhat arbitrary division of humans into five levels of health, to be described shortly. As you read on, see where you and your family fit in this picture, and consider what you might safely do to move your whole family up into a more comfortable, disease-free existence.

At the top level a person is at peak efficiency and well-being. At the fifth level he is sick enough to be hospitalized— on intravenous fluids, three medicines, an antibiotic or two, maybe oxygen, even catheters. We all know what the sixth level would be. Most of us live on the second to fourth levels, often going up to a higher level but unable to remain for long in an enhanced state of health.

Sliding down through the levels is all too easy if a combination of stresses and unlucky events occurs. Consider a baby, nine months of age, who has cut four teeth (a stress). His mother decides to stop nursing him (a stress). He develops a cold. In four days he has 102° fever and an earache (a stress). His doctor gives him a shot of ampicillin (a stress). After taking additional medicine orally for five days he develops diarrhea (a stress). His appetite is off (a stress). He can only drink sugar water (a stress). He seems symptom-free for three weeks (no stress). The weather changes or his babysitter sneezes on him; he gets a fresh cold (a stress). He gets another ear infection, this time accompanied by a febrile convulsion—a real stress. He gets a spinal tap, more antibiotics, and is placed on phenobarbital to prevent a recurrence.

He has gone from perfect health (Level I) to Level III in six short weeks. Prophylactic medicines prescribed by the doctor will keep him from Level IV (tubes in ears, adenoidectomy, allergy tests). A stress-free period of recovery and proper care should bring him back to Level I.

These levels are not clear-cut. Health states are a continuum; one thing leads to another—for better or worse. The more you sink, the more the doctor is required. The better you maintain your body, the less likely you are to experience bouts of illness.

Your family doctor can tell you what you need to know about the biochemistry and genetic predispositions of your family. Armed with this knowledge, you will be able to follow an individualized program of nutrition and preventive maintenance, so each of you can live at an optimum level of health.

Level I

This infant grows to adulthood free of illness, rashes, gas, headaches, fatigue, depression, insomnia. He* came from a stress-free, comfortable, full-term pregnancy and easy delivery. He laughs and smiles more than he cries and frowns. His hair and nails are glossy, not brittle, require a minimum of care, and his scalp is smooth and clean. His bowel movements have an acid odor with little or no putrid, nauseating smell. He's never constipated (well, hardly ever) nor does he have loose, sloppy, green BMs. He does not bruise easily nor can one raise a wheal easily by scratching his skin. When he cries his nose runs clear; he breathes easily with no hyponasal twang to his voice. He sneezes, snores, and coughs rarely. No blood is noticed from his nose unless injured, and then it stops quickly.

He cuts teeth easily. He handles weather changes, teething, going to school, learning new skills, athletic exertion, and other stresses with a minimum of psychosomatic symptoms. He can eat many foods and occasionally even junk food or sugar without a headache or fainting or fatigue. His permanent teeth are even, free of cavities, uncrowded, and there is room for his wisdom teeth. No orthodontia is needed.

He is likely to come from a family that seems calm and accepting. There is little or no obesity, diabetes, allergy, alcoholism, schizophrenia, or depression in his family background. He is more likely than not to be brown-eyed (American Indians excepted) and he tans easily.

He works up to his ability in school, is not easily distracted, learns to read easily, finishes assigned work, is usually compliant and easygoing. He makes friends easily and has a

---

* The word *he*, used in these examples and throughout this book, is of course the generic use—still a kind of communication shorthand—and almost always really means "he *or* she."

pleasant personality.   He is adroit and coordinated.   He is neither thin nor fat.

He has few extremes of emotional response—he cries or laughs appropriately.   He enjoys doing things for others.

He sails through his developmental levels in physical, psychological, and cognitive growth as if he had read the charts.   He does not prolong bed-rocking, thumb-sucking, hair-twisting; he is able to abandon such behavior as he matures without fuss.   He is easy to toilet-train; he almost seems to do it himself when ready for it.

He enjoys pleasing his loved ones.   He can also entertain himself.   As he grows he can even laugh at his own human frailties.   If he experiments with drugs, it is only because his peer group suggests it; he abandons them because he finds his drug-free existence more comfortable.

He is a satisfactory, fun-to-have-around child.   A joy. He even remembers *your* birthday and anniversary.

Level II

There is nothing very wrong here, but the differences suggest a slippage that, if unchecked, could slide on down to disease and misery.   Remedial action is called for.   He still laughs more than he cries and in general is a satisfactory baby, child, adolescent, adult, parent, but he has occasional moments of allergy, discontent, moodiness, sickness.   His nose may run when he is on the wool rug for more than three hours.   He doesn't sleep through the night until three months of age. He lollygags over breast or bottle and vomits once or twice a week when handled by a stranger.   A cold develops only if someone brings it home—maybe two or three times a year— and clears rapidly with nose drops and antihistamines without accompanying ear infection.

Bouts of gas and fussiness are rare but real and are dispelled by tea, massage, or a glycerin suppository.   He is not completely satisfied on the breast and sometimes has gas if his mother eats beans, garlic, or onions. If overfed he will vomit. An occasional BM may stink.

His development matches the standard charts but he is occasionally frustrated because he crawls under a table and can't get out. He loves cuddling. He insists on sucking or rocking and needs a favorite stuffed toy at bedtime. Separation anxiety comes early—at seven or eight months—but he can be distracted out of it.

Teething may be accompanied by a fever (100° to 101°) but aspirin is curative; no disease follows. He gets roseola but is not "sick": he just feels warm and is irritable for three days and then has a body rash and resumes smiling.

He has food preferences but can be talked into eating almost everything except liver and spinach. Rashes appear (cheeks, face, buttocks) with some new foods but disappear in a day or so. He has a hard BM only with too much rice, applesauce, or bananas.

Temper tantrums are short; he gives them up when his parents turn their backs. In a month he finds better ways to express himself: "No!" He cruises about the house touching things but seems careful and looks to his parents for approval. If they say no, he understands and does not again touch the forbidden object.

He has little trouble getting toilet-trained: a few dry runs and false alarms and several accidents. Girls are trained at eighteen to twenty months and boys by two and a half to three years.

Only one attack of croup per winter and only one strep throat in every two or three years; the former is assuaged with steam in two nights and the latter responds nicely to penicillin.

School is a little scary for a day or two but when he gets his bearings he is cooperative, a leader, and has fun. He learns easily but occasionally goes off the page and writes on his neighbor. He is sorry if he hurts someone. Only a few accidents, and never suturable cuts or concussions. He is careful with toys. Never sticks a bean up his nose. He waits to ride a bike until he is sure he can, then he does it easily. Remembers danger when warned.

Enjoys sweets but has no obvious food cravings. Accepts punishment if fair. Goes to bed with only a little reluctance.

Plays cooperatively with others. Likes to win but accepts a loss cheerfully. Doesn't care if chosen fourth when sides are picked. Defends self in a fight but will not start one. Mood swings are slight and evanescent. Will not think of mean things to do to the losers in his class and joins in only reluctantly if his peer group picks on someone.

Growth is even. During ages seven to twelve he enjoys his parents as much as his friends. Invites a friend over as if proud of his home and family. Would prefer certain toys or games on birthdays but appears pleased if relatives give shirts and pajamas.

Only rarely does he awaken his parents because of nocturnal fears; may wet bed only after an exciting party or scary movie. Does his fair share of chores within twenty-four hours after the request, rarely complains that he is a slave.

Adolescence is generally smooth since he has enough supportive friends and hobbies. Only twenty pimples in six years. Never gets mononucleosis. Only an occasional stomachache if he forgets breakfast or before a big game. Good at team sports; cooperative. A few muscle cramps after exercises.

Sneezes for a week during pollen season. Gets athlete's foot but it is easily cleared with an over-the-counter fungicide. Gets sweaty palms and rapid pulse on his first date. Masturbates once or twice a week and feels guilty but doesn't lose sleep over it. Laughs when friends say he will get hair growing on his palm. Smokes off and on; enjoys beer with friends.

Level III

The mother of the child in this category usually had a stressful pregnancy: nausea and vomiting, mild toxemia, spotty bleeding, prolonged or early or Caesarean delivery. The baby may have been premature, was slow to breathe, had to go into the incubator, perhaps also needed oxygen. Because of these factors the mother and baby are not allowed to participate in early, important mother-child interaction. She may be too weak to nurse and he may be too tired to suck, so the "helpful" nursery team puts him on cow's milk and she dries up.

He picks up on weight and strength and things go well for about two to four weeks, when colic, eczema, wheeze or vomiting, gas, and diarrhea push a barely Level I baby into Level II or III. The doctor is summoned and may be able to prevent a further decline to Level IV. But these are the babies who get colic medicines, antihistamines, antibiotics, ointments, and milk changes and whose families need tranquilizers, sedatives, and aspirin.

These children are touchy, often uncuddlable—as if the world is too close. They may fight back or occasionally withdraw, suck their thumbs or rock the bed with a determination that suggests they are trying to block out a sensory overload. We want to cuddle and comfort them, but if we get too close they arch away or stiff-arm us or get so tense they will vomit—the ultimate in body language, indicating rejection of our advances.

This hypertonic baby is the one who should have been nursed, the one most likely to have come into the world with exhausted adrenal glands and, as a consequence, the one who would most likely develop an allergy to cow's milk. As noted above, one stress leads to another and he hovers between

Levels III and IV. If the parents can hold him together he may outgrow his problems, but each new stress will surely overburden his weak defenses. Repeated infections, intestinal upsets, rashes, allergies force the parents to overprotect him and make a "hothouse plant" out of him. Hypochondriasis and constant navel-gazing seem to be his lot.

He overreacts to separation; has violent temper tantrums over the slightest insult; is noncompliant in eating, toilet training. He feels put upon. Birthdays, outings, surprises are overwhelming invasions of his privacy or opportunities to become a tyrannical monster. He is accident-prone, a bull in a china shop, shows no remorse if he hurts someone, does not seem to profit by mistakes, and cannot seem to comprehend parental instruction.

He is either terribly shy or a persistent approacher—he cannot ignore unimportant stimuli. Either environmental stimuli overwhelm him and he retreats in fear or has to attack everything that appears in his environment. Everything must go his way—no compromise, no give and take—and when sick he expects to be waited on hand and foot.

He has few friends in school, but he may be the class clown. He makes the rules for the games; he needs to win and will cheat to do it. He is a Jekyll-and-Hyde type of person, showing wild swings of mood. He can be very affectionate if he wants something, pouts or storms if he gets only a fair share.

He has persistent allergies. He needs antihistamines and occasional shots of cortisone for bee stings or bad bouts of asthma or a completely plugged nose during pollen season. He is likely to have had his tonsils removed and had tubes in his ears; he may have been on prophylactic antibiotics to suppress infections. His attacks of colds usually last longer than those of his siblings and are more likely to go into secondary bacterial infection.

Intestinal flu exhausts him. He is more likely than not

to be hospitalized when sick because home nursing care never seems to be adequate. He dehydrates easily when sick.

His nights do not seem restful. He may resist going to bed. He awakens screaming with a night terror once a month, or he sleeps deeply and wets the bed. He is a grouchy bear in the morning and ruins whatever cheerful interaction his parents try to observe at breakfast. He often refuses breakfast.

You know that if he would eat properly he would feel better. It almost seems as if he enjoys feeling punk. He is sallow and usually has dark circles under his eyes. He gets head- and stomachaches easily, especially if he is asked to do a chore. He may wear a jacket when everyone else is comfortable in a shirt. When adults speak to him he sits impassively with his arms folded on his chest. He acts as if he wants people to dislike him.

Adolescence is difficult. He tries alcohol, cigarettes, and pot at eleven or twelve years of age and drugs at thirteen or fourteen. His friends are often the losers.

Acne is moderately severe and persistent. His hair is stringy or greasy. He doesn't seem to care. He has a bad self-image. Teachers don't like him and hope he will drop out of school; he hopes he will be expelled because he hates school anyway.

It takes a lot of social, parental, psychiatric, and medical help to keep him from juvenile delinquency. He could slip easily into a lifetime antisocial commitment.

Level IV

Individuals unfortunate enough to qualify for this category require almost constant medical attention: daily drug therapy for epilepsy, diabetes, cystic fibrosis; gamma globulin and antibiotics to ward off infections; weekly allergy shots; antileukemia medicines; surgery for congenital anomalies, twisted bowels, kidney malfunctions, tumors, or blood clots;

cortisone on a daily basis to control arthritis, colitis, nephritis, asthma. All attest to the seriousness of this level of trouble.

For many children, however, the bodies may have arrived at this level but the emotional and intellectual level may still be up at the I and II area. Some have bodies and general physical health that qualify them for Level I or II but their psyche is at the fourth level: depression, phobias, extreme hyperactivity, belligerence, migraine.

Level V

This category contains the bedridden, terminally ill, extremely retarded or malformed—the child about whom doctors become very depressed. We would like to help, but the conditions seem irreversible.

These levels are merely illustrative of a continuum of behavioral characteristics. Your child need not have *all* the characteristics of each level to force a label or cause needless concern. These profiles provide me with a general guide as to how heroic I must be with nutritional supports. Some children in Level II or III need only diet changes; others in Levels IV and V would more likely need high-potency vitamins, even injections in high doses to reverse the rapid slippage.   □

If school authorities want to stop discipline problems and vandalism in the classroom, they must do away with sugar and junk foods in the halls and close the candy stores within two miles of the school.

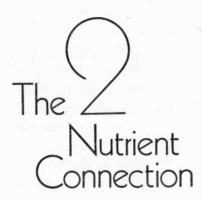

The 2 Nutrient Connection

Most of us have deficiencies in nutrients from time to time. Requirements for various foods, vitamins, and minerals vary from person to person, depending on age and sex, on the season of the year, and on individual stresses and traumas. The demands of life are variable and it is not always possible to predict and prepare for them.

The concept of optimum nutrition is based on the relationship between quantities required and quantities supplied. At no time is the average person completely deficient in a needed nutrient; the problem is usually a lack of an adequate amount. Depending upon the importance of the particular nutrient that is deficient, our bodies function less than optimally. Since some of the needed nutrients are available in the foods most of us normally eat, we know we are getting some of them. But are we getting as much as we need?

To encourage parents to use food as a supportive system of medical care, my nutrition program must be logical and fairly easy to execute—or it won't be followed. There are general considerations and also specific recommendations for specific symptoms. The credo is "a specific treatment for a specific disease," but we recognize that most tissues of the body require many varying nutrients to make them function properly; for example, skin health usually requires zinc, vitamin A, and the B complex. Thus the program aims at supplying nutrients in the right combinations and amounts to correct the patient's particular problem.

It is, however, useless to attempt to try specific supplements when a brief review of the patient's eating habits reveals that he is consuming large quantities of antinutrients. What's an antinutrient? It is a substance that, when consumed, in and of itself increases the body's need for more nutrients. (*See* Chapter 3.) Examples: refined sugar, excessive carbohydrates, artificial additives. Many times the mere elimination of the antinutrients will be all the help the body needs to raise it from one level to the next higher level (assuming that the antinutrients are replaced by wholesome food).

In no way do I imply—nor should any reader interpret—that the services of the medical doctor should be avoided; he is knowledgeable and eager to diagnose and treat the problem, especially if it is a life-threatening disease. But once you have found your child's level and have determined the nutritional deficiencies, you should make some adjustment in diet and lifestyle or you will certainly be back in his office.

Children usually hate vitamins because the B vitamins, especially, taste like moldy dirt. Using cod-liver oil drops from early infancy might be a good way to start, rather than introducing it to the negative two-year-old. Brewer's yeast and wheat germ mixed in with old-fashioned peanut butter or fruit is a useful suggestion. Vitamin C comes as a concentrated powder that can be stirred into juices. Calcium and magnesium come as powdered dolomite, which tastes like chalk.

If one can banish antinutrients and get the whole family on a program of sound nutrition, within three or four weeks everybody should feel better and be more cheerful. Persistent rashes and watery noses should clear up. Head- and stomach-aches should be gone or be only mild. Tempers will not flare so easily. It is important that the whole family follow good eating habits. If father still puts sugar in his coffee and has a piece of pie for dessert in front of the five-year-old who loves pie but gets six grapes and a piece of cheese instead, the program will break down.

Try the new or increased amounts of the nutrients. Be persistent. Give each change a month or two. You have the ultimate responsibility for the health of yourself and your spouse and children. If you and your child are still sickly or not feeling well, get a good checkup and a diagnosis from a reliable internist, family-practice specialist, or pediatrician. (I am assuming if you had something awful, you would have been there two or three months earlier.)

If everything checks out all right—no infection, no surgical condition—it would be smart to seek out a doctor who is nutrition-oriented, whether a chiropractor, a naturopath, or a dentist. So-called orthomolecular doctors practice on the theory that if all the cells of the body are nourished properly, the body should be able to withstand a rather hostile environment—that is, stress and all its subdivisions, including infections, injuries, emotional traumata, and (up to a point) nutritional deprivations. Biochemistry has now advanced to the state where all the important chemicals needed by the body and present in foods are known.

The important variables that often make the services of a skilled nutrition-oriented therapist necessary are: (1) The food one eats; although carefully selected, it may not have its full complement of vitamins and minerals because of processing or growth in inferior soil; (2) a digestive mechanism that may be unable to absorb everything the individual eats; (3) genetic factors that cause one person to need a specific nutrient in amounts several times greater than the average; (4) a family history in which the mother (and perhaps the father) was not nourished properly prior to conception or birth.

If a patient has really tried to get better—has taken vitamin shots, has fasted* for a few days, has seen two or three doctors who suggest psychotherapy (which can help)—but has not improved, I order a hair analysis. The results will indicate if there is overingestion or underingestion or improper storage of one or more of fifteen to eighteen minerals and will tell something about exposure to poisonous heavy metals. A blood test for these elements is a good idea, but the body in its effort to create homeostasis will keep these important nutrients at a fairly consistent level even though some sacrifice is made (such as pulling calcium out of calcium-poor bones to keep the blood calcium constant).

There is no reason you cannot lift yourself and your family out of your present level and enjoy the fun of sound health, the feeling of exhilaration on awakening cheerfully in the morning, the excitement of new experiences.

The majority of symptoms that present themselves are the result of deficiencies in one or more of the various members of the vitamin B complex. Being water-soluble, these vitamins do not tend to accumulate in the body, yet they are so intimately involved in the body's biochemistry that when trouble occurs it is the B vitamins that most frequently are the culprits.

At this point it will be useful to take a look at the various vitamins and minerals the body needs for healthy functioning.

---

* *Fasting* must be supervised by an interested physician. Usually plenty of fluids (tea or vegetable juice) and C and B vitamins are given to keep the patient from dehydrating. In about four to five days, if the patient feels renewed, cheerful, and symptom-free, it suggests he was eating something to which he was allergic (usually his favorite food).

The guidelines that follow are brief. Try to commit them to memory. They will give you an understanding of the essential nutrients, some of the ways they interrelate, and some of the best food sources for obtaining them.

In composing menus for family meals, keep this in mind: If the family feels better or is less sick after experimenting with vitamins and minerals, try to concentrate on the foods that contain the beneficial nutrient. For example, if vitamin C in large doses is helpful for colds and allergies, foods high in vitamin C should be emphasized daily. You may find that the supplements can be reduced as time goes by.

Food and Vitamin Guide

If one suspects a deficiency of the following vitamins or minerals, it would be worthwhile to ingest a concentrated form of the missing nutrient for four to six weeks and then try to use the food or herb that is known to be high in that substance —probably for life. If the symptoms or signs recur, it suggests that the body has higher than normal requirement for that vitamin or mineral and the concentrate is also required in the higher than usually recommended amount. We are all different, and each of us must find his own specific requirement, not just for survival, which is the value of the Recommended Daily Allowance (RDA), but for optimum health.

Vitamin A is necessary for skin and membrane function, skeletal development, and good vision. Stress or infection to those tissues would suggest increasing the daily dose. 15,000 to 30,000 units is about right for most of us. (RDA is only 5000 units per day.) If skin is dry and feels like a nutmeg grater and there is a susceptibility to respiratory infection and cavities, vitamin A should be increased. Vitamin E, B_2, and zinc make the A work on tissues better. Bile salts, lecithin, and fats are necessary for the A to be absorbed. Unconcentrated cod liver oil may be the best.

Respiratory, skin, eye, ear infections, colitis, gastritis, and genital infections all use up large amounts of A. Stress lowers protein and, since protein carries A to the tissues, protein and A must be increased during sickness and stress. Excessive menstrual flow may suggest a low level of A; double it for a month or add vitamin E to increase the efficiency of the A. Increased amounts of 50,000 to 150,000 units would be needed if there is constant eye use or strain, psoriasis, warts, eczema, gum disease, or alcoholism. (Infants should not get more then 20,000 units.)

The liver turns carotene into vitamin A. Carotene is plentiful in endive and the greens of dandelions, spinach, turnips, beets, lettuce, parsley. Carrots, sweet potatoes, squash, apricots, and peaches are good. Liver, eggs, and some dairy products are high in vitamin A content. (Certified raw milk comes from better-fed cows.)

B complex vitamins are important for the conversion of foods to energy. Nerve tissue, skin, hair, eyes, mouth, and the liver especially need the B vitamins to function optimally. And increased amounts are necessary for the stress of emotional trauma, infection, and during pregnancy and growth. Although they all should be taken together and best at mealtimes, each of the Bs has been found to have some specific effects. Good sources are brewer's yeast, wheat germ, fish, meat (especially liver), nuts.

B_1, or thiamine, seems to be a nervous system equalizer, cheering the depressed, energizing the fatigued, calming the hyperactive; good for morale and in helping to control emotions. A B_1 deficiency lowers thyroid function, causes loss of appetite, is seen in digestive disturbances, and can cause in-

crease in pain and noise sensitivity. B_1 is most plentiful in pork, beef heart, and avocados. Most legumes and nuts have a fair amount. B_1 minimum is 2 mg per day but up to 100 mg per day for a while may be necessary to correct a deficiency. Increased amounts are needed to counteract the effects of alcoholism, anemia, constipation or diarrhea (or indigestion in general), nausea, stress, rapid heart beat.

B_2, or riboflavin, aids vitamin A in controlling skin disorders (cracks about mouth, gritty sensation of eyelids, eye fatigue, and light sensitivity). Eczema may be calmed with B_2, probably because it is needed by the adrenals to produce cortisol. B_2 daily needs begin at 2 mg (RDA), but up to 100 mg per day might be necessary. Acne, alcoholism, arthritis, diabetes, any digestive disturbance, and, of course, stress would require these increased amounts. B_2 is abundant in cheese, eggs, and oysters.

B_3, or niacinamide, seems to elevate the depression due to hypoglycemia; those who suddenly stop eating sugar will find B_3 helps during the withdrawal phase. B_3 may increase energy levels and control some headaches. It may also improve concentration. B_3 daily intake should be at least 20 mg (RDA), but some people require 200 to 500 mg a day. Some schizophrenics can be helped with up to 3000 mg a day. It may improve appetite loss, control canker sores, headaches, and even halitosis. B_3 needs are elevated in stress, indigestion, leg cramps, and tooth decay. Seafood and dairy products are high in niacin. B_3 is also found in legumes, mushrooms, fish, fowl, and pork.

B_6, or pyridoxine, has been used for adrenal gland exhaustion. It improves conditions for which cortisone drugs might be indicated (hay fever, asthma, and auto-immune diseases). It may prevent the premenstrual symptoms of acne,

irritability, depression, and headache, as it allows the liver to metabolize female hormones. It is also a safe diuretic and may prove dramatic for the morning nausea and vomiting of pregnancy. Anxiety and craving for sweets can be stopped with extra B_6 (50 to 200 mg per day). It is known to improve memory, so dyslexia victims might profit from this. Nocturnal aches and stiffness in hands, fingers, and feet may respond to B_6. Oily scales, cradle cap, and dandruff on scalp, brows, and eyelids may disappear with B_6. Three days of B_6 before a trip may prevent seasickness. B_6 intake should be at least 2 mg a day (RDA) but under the special situations mentioned above, up to 100 to 400 mg per day may be required. Some infantile convulsions may be stopped with B_6. It is found in brewer's yeast, meat, whole grains, and leafy vegetables.

Pantothenic acid is a cortisone precursor and along with the other Bs, vitamin A, and C should improve an allergy problem, regardless of its cause. From 100 mg up to 3000 mg a day may be used. It can be effective against canker sores, if big doses are started early enough. RDA is only 10 mg. Most intestinal disorders, including duodenal ulcers, may be helped. Allergic skin (eczema) and respiratory (asthma) problems may be attenuated. Some cases of alopecia areata (*see* p. 47) may clear up. A week of 200–500 mg of pantothenic acid a day may ease sore and aching muscles. Some forms of arthritis may respond to large doses. Pantothenic acid is in fair supply in legumes, mushrooms, eggs, broccoli, cauliflower, pork, and beef.

Folic acid is considered a blood builder. Only small amounts are needed. A lack of this may lead to fatigue, insomnia, constipation, and restless legs. Folic acid may mask a pernicious anemia produced by a B_{12} deficiency. As much as 0.1 mg is usually easily obtained from food; a prescription

is necessary for the 1 mg size. RDA is 400 mcg. (0.4 mg).
Some bodies may require 10 mg or more, especially in some
forms of anemia, growth problems, alcoholism, stress, mental
problems, and stomach ulcers. If the concentrated pill or shot
is helpful, the diet should be increased in amounts of green
leafy vegetables, fresh cow's milk, organ meats, and whole
grains. (Dates and tuna fish have high amounts.)

B_{12} is essential for blood also, and is found in animal
protein, so vegetarians usually need to take a supplement. A
shot of B_{12} will sometimes stop postpartum depression overnight. Only 5 micrograms (RDA) should be enough, but 100
to 1000 micrograms occasionally may be necessary to get someone out of a nutritional hole. B_{12} shots might be helpful to
control allergies, fatigue, insomnia, shingles, stress, and appetite loss. Blood-cell formation and a healthy nervous system
require B_{12}. Fatigue and weakness are frequently improved
dramatically with B_{12}; doctors should not be embarrassed to
treat "hypochondriasis" with B_{12} shots, as this illness is frequently an undiagnosed B_{12} deficiency.

Biotin needs are easily derived from plants and animal
foods. Biotin is manufactured by the intestinal bacteria in
good amounts, so oral antibiotics, which tend to kill all bacteria
in the body indiscriminately, might reduce the supply. If the
vitamin bottle label says about 100 to 500 micrograms, it
should be adequate. Extra amounts, up to 1,000 (1.0 mg),
may be worthwhile for dry skin, eczema, and baldness.

Inositol is easy to obtain from almost any food and a
vitamin supplement may be redundant, but 1000 mg would
do well. It is worth adding to the supplements if hair loss is
the problem. It is involved in lecithin metabolism, so in families with cholesterol elevation foods with increased amounts

would be worthwhile. Citrus fruits, meat, milk, nuts, and brewer's yeast are good sources.

Para-amino benzoic acid (*PABA*) as a lotion is an effective sun screen and has been used to restore color to gray hair. Ten to 50 mg a day internally should be enough and is usually obtained with any fairly good diet. This amount along with other B vitamins should help fatigue, constipation, depression, headaches, and irritability. Sizable amounts are found in organ meats, brewer's yeast and wheat germ.

Choline is usually found in B supplements but is more of a food, and is easily supplied by any reasonably good diet.

Whole grains, brewer's yeast, and liver are all good sources of B and obviously more complete than taking each B as a separate supplement. A few teaspoonsful of brewer's yeast in a baby's diet each day can change a thin, weak, pale, irritable infant into a smiling, pink-cheeked, hungry, active, fun-to-show-off-to-relatives baby.

Vitamin C seems to hold the body together, detoxifies poisons, has antiviral and antihistamine properties, and is needed by the adrenal glands to produce the hormones needed to fight stress. Because we are all different in our perceptions of stress, everyone must alter his intake of vitamin C until stress appears under control—fewer colds, fewer allergies, fewer nosebleeds. The daily dose of at least 50 (RDA) to 100 mg for a reasonably normal child should be increased by a factor of 5 to 10 times in anticipation of stress (trip, visit, party, holiday, school, immunizations, exposure to disease or prodromal symptoms of anything). Diarrhea would suggest that one has reached one's tolerance. With some persons, canker sores may result from use of vitamin C; in which case sodium ascorbate might be tried.

It probably works better if taken with rutin and bio-flavenoids. (These are found in the white pulp of citrus fruits.) Oranges, grapefruit are good sources, but don't forget parsley, green peppers, mustard greens, and watercress. Other vitamin C deficiency signs are a tendency toward bruising easily, dental caries, touchy gums, and poor digestion. Vitamin C by pill or foods with high concentration of C should be given to those with infections, hepatitis, sinusitis, arthritis, allergies, cystitis, and stress.

Vitamin D is fat-soluble, so it will be stored in the body and could be toxic. Sunlight on the skin is the safest way for the body to manufacture this, but fish-liver oil is the best assur-ance if sunlight is unreliable (northern climes or when the sun is screened out by pollution). 400 (RDA) to 1500 units seem about right as a daily dose. It would be wise to increase the dose of D and calcium and phosphorus (bone meal) after a fracture or bone injury and, of course, during periods of extra need: rapid growth in infancy, adolescence and pregnancy and lactation.

Vitamin E, or tocopherol, has been described as a scav-enger, as it has the ability of combining with and rendering harmless many pollutants and chemicals in the food, air and water. It is also an anti-oxidant. It has been used to reduce varicose veins, hemorrhoids, the pain of exercise cramps, rectal cramps, menstrual cramps, and the pain of burns (when locally applied). It calms restless legs. It may prove valuable in the premature to protect against retrolental fibroplasia (*see* p. 94) and some of the lung immaturity to which these infants are prone. As it reduces the clumping of platelets it is considered important as a prophylaxis against clogged blood vessels. It makes for increased effectiveness of vitamin A. It should be increased with increase in exercise; and is best not given with iron.

Children should get 200 units daily and adults 400 units or more. It is natural in many foods, especially whole grains, nuts, and legumes. Mixed tocopherols is the preferred form. The RDA is a paltry 15 IU.

Vitamin K is easily manufactured by intestinal bacteria, and thus would only be needed as a supplement at birth before these bacteria have been established or after oral antibiotics that could interfere with the bacterial synthesis of this blood-coagulation vitamin.

Fatty acids are usually manufactured by the body if there is some fat in the diet, but some essential acids must be provided. Dry skin, eczema, brittle hair and nails, or weight problems may suggest a deficiency. Wheat germ, sunflower seeds, safflower, corn, or soy oils supply these. Two percent milk is better than skim milk for this objective.

Calcium is required all our lives for bones, teeth, muscle and nerve function, and for blood clotting. A quart of milk has about 1000 mg, which is about the right daily dose. Pasteurization decreases the availability of calcium to the body—which may explain why so many children who consume large amounts of milk have low levels of calcium in their hair and become calmer, sleep better, and have fewer muscle cramps when dolomite, bone meal, or calcium tablets are added to the diet. A possible explanation may be that an allergy to the milk protein somehow prevents the absorption of the calcium through the intestinal wall when these two nutrients are present simultaneously.

The prudent pregnant woman should ingest about 2 grams of calcium a day, especially if she cannot tolerate dairy products. The bones store calcium under the influence of vitamin D and hormones regulate the calcium level in the blood by releasing or redepositing the calcium as necessary.

The blood calcium may not give an accurate clue as to a deficiency or overload in the body; a hair assay might be revealing.

Muscle pains, cramps, twitches, and even convulsions may suggest a calcium deficiency. Menstrual cramps, "charley-horses" and shin splints suggest the need for calcium. Some hyperactive children are safely calmed with calcium; they sleep better and handle stress better with a calcium supplement. Vitamin C helps in the absorption of calcium. The American diet contains a lot of phosphorus (meat, cereal, soft drinks); the ideal ratio of calcium to phosphorus in the diet is about three to two. Cutting down the amount of phosphorus and increasing the calcium intake should improve this ratio.

Infants should receive about 800 to 1000 mg of calcium; rapidly growing adolescents about 1500 mg, and pregnant and lactating mothers about 2000 mg. Milk may not be the perfect food, so dolomite (two parts calcium to one part magnesium) or bone meal (a source of phosphorus) might be best. Cod-liver oil should probably be taken close to the time of calcium ingestion.

Calcium is also found in nuts, legumes, sardines, oysters, soy beans, wheat germ, cabbage, and turnip greens. Calcium helps to displace lead from tissues and bones; a good daily supply of calcium may prevent this common pollutant from becoming a personal problem. (Don't use bone meal from old English horses; many have much lead in their bones.)

Arthritis victims usually have demineralized bones so calcium supplements are wise. Many pregnant women take 1000 to 2000 mg of some calcium source just prior to delivery and notice decrease in pain but not in the force of labor.

Magnesium is also needed for teeth and bones but its action is more especially related to the nervous tissue reactivity. If the level of magnesium is low one becomes apprehensive, excitable, and may have muscle twitches or convulsions that are not responsive to calcium. Cow's milk, meat, and eggs are low in magnesium; the higher the protein intake, the more magnesium is required, as it activates a number of enzymes involved in the metabolism of most foods ingested.

Magnesium has a regulating or calming effect; it has been beneficial for the hyperactive, restless child. Along with B_6 it may improve his memory, reduce his "goosiness" and startle reaction. It can fight the fatigue that accompanies nervous exhaustion.

Teeth and bones are stronger if magnesium accompanies the calcium; calcium seems to need magnesium. Some persons find that they do better if half the daily calcium comes from bone meal and the other half from dolomite. Probably 250 to 600 mg of magnesium a day is about right, but if the stools tend to be sloppy this may be cut back. The bedwetter who cannot hold more than 3 or 4 ounces of urine without jumping up and down may be helped in just a few days with magnesium.

Magnesium helps to prevent kidney-stone formation as a diet low in magnesium lets more calcium go to the kidneys. Magnesium, in some, has a relaxing effect on the blood-vessel muscles (might lower high blood pressure).

Magnesium is involved with the control of cell membrane electrical charge and, of course, with the nutriments getting into the cells. Magnesium may help the stressed person to cope; it filters out some extraneous stimuli. It is found in kelp and seafoods, nuts, whole grains, green vegetables, and apricots, figs, and dates.

Phosphorus is abundant in wheat germ, seeds, nuts, and meats. It requires the presence of calcium and vitamin D for proper utilization, and should be taken in slightly smaller amounts than the calcium. Bone meal is a good source.

Iron is essential for the manufacture of red blood cells. Iron-deficiency anemia is a common ailment in infants and young children because of rapid growth and large milk (usually cow's) intake. If a nursing mother is eating nutritious foods, her baby will get enough iron from the milk and may not need an iron tonic or iron-bearing foods to prevent anemia. But the rapid growth of the prematurely born baby plus the fact that his early birth cheated him from getting much iron in his storage depots make iron supplementation mandatory. In years past solid foods were introduced early to preclude the development of this anemia, but the risk of a carbohydrate and salt load and food allergies now make it wise to start solids— one new food a month—after six to eight months of age. But the prematurely born infant should probably have some iron drops daily after age three months.

Inorganic iron (ferrous salts) is poorly tolerated; diarrhea or constipation may result, so organic sources are best. Liver, meats, brewer's yeast, wheat germ, eggs, seeds, almonds, parsley, prunes, raisins, and leafy vegetables are all good sources for the older child. Molasses contains iron but we try to discourage too much reliance on sweets.

About 15 to 25 mg of iron a day is a good target—more, of course, for menstruating and pregnant women. But only about 10 to 20 percent of iron is absorbed. Vitamin C aids iron absorption. B_6, folic acid, cobalt, copper, and B_{12} are needed to put the hemoglobin molecule together. Desiccated liver is a good source for everything needed to do this. (Some authorities even suggest cooking things in iron pots.)

Zinc is essential for a number of important functions. Zinc deficiency may account for eczema, acne, dwarfism, poor wound healing, white spots in the nails, and small testicles. Alcohol will remove zinc from the liver and it may be lost in the urine. Sperm has the highest percent of zinc of any cell in the body; infertility in males may be due to a lack or loss of zinc. (Alcoholic males are frequently infertile.) An inflamed prostate may be due to low zinc levels. Also, low levels of zinc may cause fatigue and decreased alertness.

Zinc is present in insulin and is a factor in at least 25 enzymes that do the work of the body: in the synthesis of nucleic acid, DNA, skin protein formation (hence the benefit for acne victim), adrenal gland function, taste bud activity and production of many of the brain's chemicals. Zinc may reduce the ravages of stomach and duodenal ulcers, regional enteritis, rheumatoid arthritis, and many stress-related diseases. Low levels of zinc may be found in those susceptible to infection. Zinc may stop body odors.

Zinc and copper have a reciprocal relationship. High copper levels and low zinc levels may be seen in some schizophrenics. High zinc levels, however, may decrease the copper with a possible anemia as a result. Zinc affects other vitamins too. For example, extra zinc may be needed if calcium intake is high; zinc needs vitamin A to function properly; zinc is involved with the function of the B vitamins. The body needs some of all the minerals. If they are supplied sufficiently and naturally, it usually takes what it needs and lets the rest go on through.

It is usually easy to get the minimum of 15 mg (RDA) of zinc in a diet that contains whole grains, seeds, brewer's yeast, liver, meat, and nuts. But 50 to 100 mg per day may be needed for a few weeks or months to correct a deficiency. Oysters are especially high in zinc, hence their reputation for improving fertility.

Manganese has recently been found to be insufficient in some epileptics; added manganese (20 mg per day) has reduced the frequency of convulsions in many of those with low levels. This mineral helps to control an abnormal response to sugar ingestion. In animals a low level can cause poor coordination and tremors. Soil studies show a gradual depletion. High phosphorus intake increases the need for manganese.

Five mg of manganese would be a good place to start. It should be easily obtained from wheat germ, seeds, legumes, and nuts. Buckwheat is a good source, but much depends on the availability of manganese in the soil.

Copper works with iron to make hemoglobin. Copper helps in the utilization of vitamin C. We need only about 2 mg a day but some people are getting far too much because of the use of copper tubing carrying the water supply. (An excess may cause psychosis.) Seafood, nuts, liver, and legumes should supply enough. The copper from these organic sources will not cause copper poisoning.

Chromium activates the enzymes needed in glucose metabolism. Less insulin may be required to control high blood sugar if an adequate level of chromium is present. Chromium seems to be deficient in our soil; one study indicated an increase in crop yield when chromium was added to the fertilizer. A milligram of chromium daily may be enough. Brewer's yeast, liver, wheat germ, rye, and green pepper are good sources.

Iodine, if absent from the diet, will lead to a goiter and decreased thyroid function. Iodized salt has cut down on this condition, but kelp and seafoods should supply the 0.15 mg per day needed. If oral temperature is below 97.5° on awakening in the morning and fatigue is a consistent symptom, extra iodine may improve the function of the thyroid gland.

Sodium, as in table salt, is present in abundance in foods, so the saltcellar should not be on the table. A teaspoon (4 to 5 grams) per day is easily ingested in the average diet. Excess sodium can lead to hypertension, and it also tends to push potassium out of the body. A craving for salt suggests that the craver is under stress or is deficient in a vitamin or mineral and is "looking" for it. Within a week of supplemental vitamins and minerals the salt lover will usually not need to salt food. (Low zinc levels make food seem tasteless.) Vegetarians (and cows) usually require more sodium because vegetables are low in sodium and high in potassium. Meat is already salty and should not be salted. Avoid salted nuts, potato and corn chips, canned meats and soups, and crackers. High salt intake can trigger migraine, seizures, and nervous tension.

Potassium inside the cells balances the sodium on the outside of the cells. It is necessary for proper cell functioning; muscles are weak without it. Diuretics, salt, sugar, stress, and cortisone drugs will flush it out of the body. The digestive tract needs potassium to function; low potassium can cause colic, constipation, fatigue, irritability, listlessness, and depression. High environmental heat leads to potassium loss, and salt tablets may make it worse. The body should get more potassium than sodium.

Nuts, seeds, and fruits are high in potassium; meats, olives, and cheese are high in sodium. Kelp is high in both but has more potassium. An intake of 1 to 5 grams of potassium per day is about right; less than that amount of sodium should be tried for.

Selenium, sulfur, molybdenum, cobalt, and some other trace elements are required but are usually included in the diet if the above-mentioned foods are eaten every few days. The intake would vary depending on the concentration in the soil in which the foods grew and the type of cooking used. (Steaming is best.)   □

A poor sense of humor may be the first clue of a vitamin B$_3$ (niacin, niacinamide) deficiency.

The 3 Prevention Diet

Throughout this book, you will see references to the Prevention Diet. This refers to general eating patterns every one should follow as part of a lifetime program of good nutrition. Where specific recommendations for specific illnesses are given, these are to be followed *in addition to* the Prevention Diet.

1. Avoid the antinutrients. Among the sweet foods, these include white sugar, brown sugar, even corn or cane syrup, maple syrup, molasses, and honey (some people continue the latter two items for a while, but their use should be minimal); commercial ice cream; boxed cereal (instead, use only whole-grain cereals—it is best to grind your own); white flour (enriched is not good enough—grind your own or don't bake). Avoid as many commercial products as possible. Stop homogenized, pasteurized milk for one month. If a food has been packaged, processed, added to, stabilized, emulsified, colored, or preserved, you know it is out of nature's hands. Read labels. These antinutrients require B complex vitamins in order to become digested and metabolized. If the B vitamins are not thus provided, the body will use the B vitamins destined for use in other organs, or will be unable to metabolize food completely or properly. Soon a deprived organ will fall ill because of this lack.

The antinutrients tend to cause a rapid rise in the blood sugar. Usually the pancreas responds by overproducing insulin and the blood-sugar level falls; this can cause the sensitive person to become antisocial or develop depression or a variety of psychosomatic symptoms from allergies to arthritis. In general, sugar and "junk" food, when consumed without accompanying vitamins and minerals as found in the natural state, will deplete the body until sickness waves a flag that the body has had it.

2. Eat natural foods four to six times a day, small amounts frequently. Raw vegetables are best but steam cooked or stir fried (Chinese wok method) are satisfactory. Eggs are okay because the lecithin helps metabolize the cholesterol—unless one has the rare condition of hyperlipoproteinemia, a rare genetic trait manifested by the inability to metabolize fats and cholesterol. (Have your doctor check your cholesterol if you like eggs.) Marbled beef may be dangerous (vegetarians seem to have a better longevity score than do beef-eaters); eat it only occasionally.

White cheeses (jack, Swiss, mozzarella) are preferable because of lack of coloring. Nuts, especially almonds or peanuts, are good nibbling foods because they are almost complete proteins (they have all the needed amino acids*) and can be eaten raw or as butter (make your own nut butters; avoid commercial varieties). Fish and chicken (if possible, buy chickens that have been running around pecking at seeds in a

---

* Amino acids are the building blocks of protein. Some are essential and must be ingested almost daily.

farmyard or a garden). Legumes such as peas, beans, and lentils are both nutritious and inexpensive; refrying makes them less gaseous. Fruits should be eaten raw, but because of the carbohydrate content they should be eaten with some protein: for instance, an apple with cheese, raisins with peanuts, dates with almonds. Dentists tell us children drink too many "liquid calories" and hence do not develop good jaws. Instead of apple juice, eat the apple; instead of orange juice, eat the orange (including the white membrane, to get bioflavenoids).

This diet should give you a more even feeling of energy, a desire to get out of bed in the morning, and a more cheerful demeanor. Allow it about three weeks to work. Bowel movements should be pasty, maybe even a little sloppy. Urination should take place three to five times a day.

It has been estimated that daily protein intake should be close to 2 grams of complete protein per kilogram of weight for the growing child and about 1 to 1.5 grams per kilogram for adults. This comes out to be about an ounce of good, complete protein a day for a 30-pound three-year-old.

3. Begin daily vitamins (which are really concentrated foods), assuming you and/or your children are behind in your requirements.

- Vitamins: A, 5000–10,000 units. D, 400–1000 units. C, 100–500 mg. E, 200–400 units. B complex, 25–50 mg of each of the Bs. (The label should say: B_1, 25 mg. B_2, 25 mg. B_3 (niacinamide), 25 mg. B_6 (pyridoxine), 25 mg. B_{12}, 25 mcg. Inositol, 25 mg. Choline, 25 mg. PABA, 25 mg. Pantothenic acid, 25 mg. Biotin, 250 mcg. Folic acid, 400 mcg.)
- Minerals: Calcium, 500–1000 mg. Magnesium, 250–500 mg. Zinc, 15 mg. Iodine, 0.1 mg. Copper, 1.0 mg. Manganese, 5 mg.

The Stress Formula

Stress can be an exciting challenge to some and puts others in bed with a migraine or asthma or fever. Stress comes in many forms: emotional, allergic, surgical, physical, ecological. When a person perceives stress of any kind, the blood sugar falls, which signals the adrenal glands to secrete cortisol and adrenalin. Exhausted adrenal glands, if not adequately resupplied with all the proper nutrients, will allow some genetic or familial trait to surface as an illness. When an allergy appears, for example, it suggests that the adrenal glands have not supplied the body with enough cortisol.

Another factor that makes for adrenal gland exhaustion is the inefficient screening out of the victim's environment. He may perceive a stress where the majority of his peers would feel comfortable. The world is too close and even threatening. The cortex of the brain reacts to overwhelming stimuli that other parts of the nervous system allowed to get through. The cortex assumes that attack is imminent and sends an SOS to the pituitary, which sends an instruction to the adrenals to pour out their hormones to prepare the body for fight or flight.

What a waste! If stress cannot be avoided and if the diet is inadequate to build up the glands again, the stressed body becomes the victim of a psychosomatic disease, the type and location depending on genetic factors. Hay fever, asthma, colitis, arthritis, depression, hyperactivity, and susceptibility to infections could be the manifest evidence of an inability to handle stress because of a poor system for filtering incoming stimuli, an overresponsive or sensitive cortex, low blood sugar, and exhausted adrenal glands. Once the disease is established and the diagnosis is made, the symptoms of the illness can be alleviated, but some effort must be directed to the nutrition of the adrenals, the pancreas, the liver, and, of course, the brain, to remedy the inadequacy that allowed this sequence to get started in the first place.

We know how to build up these glands so that they can function properly, but we must alter the victim's diet and life-style to prevent a recurrence of the exhaustion. The program for adrenal support therapy, called the Stress Formula throughout our text, is as follows:

- Eat no sugar, white flour, packaged cereals, or the like.
- Nibble nutritious foods every two to three hours so the blood sugar is maintained as evenly as possible. (*See* p. 30 and Afterword)
- Vitamin C, 500 to 10,000 mg per day.
- Vitamin B complex, 50 to 200 mg of each of the Bs per day for a month or so, then a lower dose perhaps for life.
- Pantothenic acid, 500 to 3000 mg per day. This can be varied up or down, depending on the severity of the allergy or other adrenal-related illness.
- Pyridoxine, B_6, in doses of 200 to 500 mg per day.
- Vitamin A, 30,000 to 50,000 units per day for a month.
- Calcium, as dolomite or bone meal or a calcium salt, in doses up to 1000 mg per day.

Some doctors find they must give vitamin C and B complex injections to supply the glands with the wherewithal to put out their valuable secretions while waiting for the glands to function efficiently. It is important to build up the glands, if there is time, so that reliance on cortisone is not necessary. Cortisone replacement may be life-saving, but because it causes a suppression of the already exhausted glands, it may be difficult to get the patient off the drug. The whole concept of adjunctive therapy is to supply the missing ingredients so the body can effectively handle *living*.

Antibiotics, tranquilizers, muscle relaxers, anticonvulsants, decongestants, antiwheeze medicines, antidepressants, and antispasmodics are all helpful but temporary, stop-gap measures. They work quickly, while the nutritional support program may take days or weeks to effect control, albeit more safely and probably more permanently. Side effects of medicines are numerous and frequently stress-producing in themselves. Since medicines are foreign chemicals, the liver must detoxify them; this requires still further nutritional supports.

Transcendental meditation, chiropractic manipulation, acupuncture, psychotherapy, hypnosis, biofeedback, and exercise all have their advocates—but all require optimum nutrition for best results. The cortex of the brain and the adrenals must be supplied with adequate amino acids, glucose, vitamins, and minerals to carry out their functions. The best foods to accomplish this are raw vegetables, seeds, nuts, whole grains, liver, fruit, fish, fowl—all as unprocessed as possible.

Pregnancy Needs

The seed must be nourished properly or the plant will be defective in some way. We know a number of things about the beginning of life. The things we do for the unborn child will have an effect lasting his whole life. It is like the powder charge for a cannonball; if only a feeble amount of good nutrition is used, the baby will be sick or have an allergy in the first few weeks of his life. But if the pregnant woman can nourish herself maximally and avoid stress, she is more likely to launch a very content, healthy child.

It is best to space children at least two or, better, three years apart. A woman's body, even with good nutrition, does not have enough chance to get its full vitality back in less time. And just having another child in the house, perfect though he or she may be, is a stress. The incidence of allergies is certainly higher in children born within one to two years after an older sibling.

During the early months of intrauterine life, the brain cells of the baby increase numerically, so constant protein nutrition is absolutely essential or this growing nervous system may not achieve its genetic potential. This is in contrast to postnatal brain development, which is largely devoted to increasing cell size. In this phase, protein is less important; temporary interruptions can be compensated for.

Work by Dr. Tom Brewer, reported by Gail Brewer in *What Every Pregnant Woman Should Know,* indicates that an average pregnant woman should gain at least 25 to 35 pounds during pregnancy. A newly pregnant obese woman should not embark on a weight-reducing diet without very careful attention to protein and vitamin intake. Apparently, the reason doctors at one time did not want their patients to gain too much was that sudden increases in weight suggest fluid storage, or edema, which could mean the possible development of hypertension, toxemia, and convulsions. It is now known that this sequence of events is almost entirely a result of the ingestion of a low-protein diet. There is a normal increase in the volume of the blood circulating during pregnancy to serve the needs of the baby. If this increase does not carry an adequate supply of albumin (protein), then by an osmotic pressure gradient, fluid will leak into the tissues. If enough fluid gets into the brain, the tissues swell and the pregnant woman may experience headache and possibly convulsions. The answer is not to give her a diuretic (water-loss substance) but to assure an adequate protein diet. No pregnant woman should ever eat food that is not completely nutritious.

It is natural for a pregnant woman to become somewhat edematous (water-logged). At the time of delivery, this extra fluid goes to the breasts and the engorgement strongly suggests to the new mother that she should nurse her baby.

Stress can be just as devastating to a pregnant woman and her baby as an inadequate diet. If a woman says she does not feel well, is nervous, on edge, depressed, overly tired, crabby, or has frequent headaches, something is wrong and remedial action must be taken to prevent her stress from affecting her child. Her stress can exhaust *his* adrenals too. The incidence of allergies, colic, infections, and hyperactivity is high in children born from mothers who had an uncomfortable or stress-filled pregnancy. A pregnant woman must have her blood checked for severe anemia, her blood pressure taken, and an evaluation made of the stress factors present (unsympathetic husband and in-laws; other worrisome children; insufficient help, money, security). Some women can handle all these stresses if they are eating properly and adhering to the Stress Formula. Some cannot absorb these things completely, so they need a vitamin B complex injection every few days to "prime the pump." These injections are a must for pregnant women who have stress plus negative genetic factors in their family background (allergies, alcoholism, obesity, diabetes, hypoglycemia). A good diet, a supportive husband, and a sympathetic doctor may not be enough.

Children who exhibit milk allergies, ear infections, tonsils and adenoids that require removal, buck teeth, mouth breathing, underslung jaw, narrow face, and tension-fatigue syndrome are more likely than not to come from mothers who had nausea and vomiting during pregnancy. This suggests that the mother was deficient in vitamin B_6, because B_6 is often curative for the nausea and vomiting. B_6 is necessary for the optimum function of the adrenal glands and the manufacture of cortisol. It is also necessary for the liver enzyme that metabolizes estrogen.

According to Weston Price in *Nutrition and Physical Degeneration,* when a young female in a primitive tribe is married, the assumption is that she will soon become pregnant. The tribe provides her the best, most nutritious foods that can be gathered from far and near, mostly protein. These tribes know that if the baby is less than perfect he will be unable to take his place in their society. His weakness, sickness, allergy, or imperfect skeletal structure will make him a liability to the tribe, which cannot provide for infirm, defective members.

Too many of our children are sickly. We now know how to make the next generation healthy, not with access to medical care and modern drugs, but with simple, fairly inexpensive, nutritious food. If we build these babies properly, they will be bright, strong and healthy.

Minimum requirements for any pregnancy would include the nutrients listed below. If a woman's body has been insulted for months or years by junk food, she might do well to increase the vitamin dosages for a few months prior to pregnancy, if she can predict a future pregnancy. Good nutrition is important through the whole nine months, but the first few weeks are vitally important.

Nutrients for Pregnancy
- No sugar except that in fruit.
- No grains except whole grains. Two to 3 ounces of nuts and seeds a day. Whole-grain bread or cereals for calories.
- 2 ounces of good-quality protein (fish, poultry, meat, eggs, liver) four to five times a day.
- 2 to 3 ounces of cheese (unprocessed white is best) or one half to one quart of raw certified cow's or goat's milk per day (unless there are allergies).
- 2 to 3 tablespoons of oil (corn, safflower, peanut).
- Vegetables—one leafy serving (lettuce, cabbage, parsley, endive, spinach).
- One root serving (carrots, beets, parsnips, turnips), raw or slightly cooked.
- Fruit—one or two servings of apple, bananas, berries, raisins. Best eaten with nuts or seeds.
- Vitamins: A, 20,000 to 30,000 units. D, 500 to 1000 units. E, 400 to 800 units. C, 500 to 5000 mg (depending on allergies and infections). B complex, 3 to 4 tablespoons

brewer's yeast or 50 mg of each of the Bs. Folic acid, 1 mg.

- Minerals: Dolomite (usually only available in 100 to 200 mg tablets), 1000 mg calcium, 500 mg magnesium (double if subject cannot tolerate dairy products). Bone meal, 500 mg. (All this can be adjusted with dairy intake to get 1500 to 2000 mg of calcium per day.) Kelp, to get iodine, zinc 30 to 50 mg, iron 20 to 40 mg, and trace amounts of all the other minerals. (*See* pp. 30, 31 and 34.)

Anti-Infection Program

Infections in children are common, but the fact that many children sail through the growing years without a cold, sore throat, or the flu *has* to indicate that there is a difference in susceptibility among individuals. We think that this difference can be explained by at least two interrelated factors: genetic differences and nutritional imbalances. This approach would help explain why some children in a family never get the flu that is sweeping through the house, while another child who is well-protected and seemingly well-fed gets a cold with no apparent exposure. An allergy that runs in a family allows viruses to get a foothold. For example, an attack of hay fever allows the cold virus to invade the nasal-lining cells, and because the area is a good culture medium the ubiquitous bacteria begin to grow there on top of the phlegm stimulated by the virus.

Obviously, a person is stuck with his genes, but it should be easy to figure out the child's infection tendencies and take steps to compensate. If allergies are rampant on both sides of a family, the pregnant woman should fortify herself before conception (if possible) with the Stress Formula up to the point where she is comfortable, stress-free, non-nauseated, and without allergies herself. She must plan to nurse the baby for six to twelve months and, of course, she follows the nutrients for pregnancy program.

If the infant becomes sick with a fever, cold, vomiting and diarrhea, croup, wheeze, colored mucus in his eyes or nose, he has slipped into a health level that may require treatment with antibiotics from a doctor, but it also signals that some defense mechanism allowed the invasion of virus or germ. Exposure to the causative agent is a valid reason for the sickness, but only a partial reason: a nutritional inadequacy facilitated the invasion.

Many infections can be aborted if vitamin C is administered before the agent begins to overwhelm the host. The failure of ascorbic acid to be therapeutic is due largely to the fact that it is not given early enough or in big enough doses. We all have individualized needs based on genetics and prenatal diet, and we have to experiment to find out just what those needs are.

If the child even looks like he is coming down with something, or sneezes a few times, or gets that pinched look, or wants to go to bed, or gets a chill, don't wait. Consult your physician and give the child approximately the following:

- Birth to 6 months: 50–100 mg vitamin C every one to two hours for the first twenty-four hours
- 6 to 12 months: 100–200 mg every one to two hours
- 12 months to 5 years: 500 mg every one to two hours
- 6 years into adulthood: 1000 mg every hour until the infection has slowed.

Taper off the dose after a day or so when improvement is obvious, but continue big doses until all the symptoms have disappeared. If diarrhea seems to be caused by the vitamin, cut back, but remember many virus infections in children will soften their stools. Rarely does vitamin C cause blood in the urine, canker sores in the mouth, or stomachaches. Cut back to a dose that will not cause such problems—or change brands, since it is possible that some impurity is causing the response. Many doctors now use 2–10 grams of vitamin C, some B_6 (500 mg), and calcium (500 to 1000 mg) intravenously for virus infections (flu, mononucleosis, hepatitis, measles) with marked success.

Timing is essential; the longer the virus has been allowed to propagate, the more difficult it is to stop its progress. Assuming that the infection got in because that particular body did not have enough vitamin C, the infection itself acts as a stress and further depletes the vitamin C, so bigger doses may be required to control the spread. If the child is sick, an antibiotic would be appropriate to help fight the infection. When the infection is over, a reappraisal of the child's lifestyle, food intake, and vitamin supplements must be made. The disease has left the child susceptible to a repeat of the illness or may even have moved the child to the next lower health level, where he surely will be more vulnerable.

This vitamin C prevention program will not work for every infection or every child, but it seems to be a safe option. Many studies indicate that megadoses of vitamin C will at least shorten the course of many common virus infections.

Inability to prevent or attenuate these infections suggests underlying allergies (food or inhalants), low vitamin A levels, or some trouble in the child's immune system that requires investigation.

Prudent parents who do not want their children to suffer will provide nourishing food and allow no sugar or white flour in the house. They will encourage exercise, with a minimum of television watching, and avoid exposure to pollution as much as possible. To seal the whole system together, they keep the children well supplied with the vitamins that are essential to support the system against stress.

Virus infections that can be helped with vitamin C include colds, croup, hepatitis, infectious mononucleosis, measles, chicken pox, mumps, canker sores, intestinal flu, and influenza.

Bacterial infections such as otitis media, streptococcal sore throat, pneumonia, sinusitis, kidney infection, and impetigo will probably need antibiotic treatment, but good preventive nutrition can keep such infections from flaring in the first place.

□

Eat only what won't rot, and eat it before it does.

More 4
Than Skin Deep

The skin—the largest organ of the body. The first to experience environmental changes (felt as pain, heat, cold, and so on), often the first to respond to stress (with such phenomena as goosepimples, blushing, hives, and perspiration).

The skin reflects general bodily conditions. If the liver is diseased with hepatitis, cirrhosis, cancer, or obstruction, the skin will appear yellow. If the patient is anemic, the skin will be pale. If dehydration is present, the skin is dry, sunken, and inelastic. Water retention due to salt in the diet or kidney disease will produce a puffiness, especially in the eyelids where the skin is loosely attached, or in the lower legs and feet because of gravity. Blue discoloration suggests the presence of unoxygenated blood from a heart or lung disorder. Itchy skin usually suggests an allergy, and if accompanied by a rash, it is likely to be a contact rash or the result of insect bites, chicken pox, or hives. If it is an "itch that rashes," it is usually a sign of eczema, a genetic-stress condition; that is, the victim has a familial tendency to eczema and the stress of his life or the environmental conditions have allowed the condition to surface.

The skin requires good and constant nutrition to maintain its integrity. Adequate protein, water, fat, the B vitamins, and vitamins E, C, and especially A are necessary.

Although many minerals are required for normal skin function, zinc seems to be of major importance. Apparently some people require more zinc and vitamin A than others because of genetic factors. To say that 5000 units per day of vitamin A (RDA) is all that anyone should have makes no sense when signs of vitamin A deficiency are obvious. Everyone is different and everyone has his or her own requirements. (Surgeons, for example, have found that if a burn patient is given zinc—up to 100 mg per day of gluconate or chelated zinc—the burn heals in half the usual time.)

Acne was once thought to result from masturbation; if an adolescent would just get married, his skin would clear up (sometimes it worked). It is now believed that acne is the skin's response to the flood of adolescent hormones and the stresses of teen-age life. Most dermatologists feel that diet has little if anything to do with the problem and rarely suggest any change. The standard treatment is to give an oral antibiotic—usually tetracycline or erythromycin—in an effort to cut down the inflammation and infection that could lead to permanent scarring. A vitamin A acid applied locally helps to peel off the surface skin so that the oil in the follicles can escape. Pimples that become cystic usually lead to pitted scars. This distressing condition is sometimes treated by injecting cortisone into the cysts to help control the inflammation.

Level I. Obviously, perfect adolescent skin requires no change in diet or nutritional or medical therapy. However, it should be explained to these twelve- to eighteen-year-olds, by someone with influence over them, that they don't lead a charmed life, that a diet of calories without accompanying minerals and vitamins will lead eventually to some problem with skin, brain, liver, lungs, or the like. A rapidly growing youth becomes desperately hungry; quick, sugary treats make him or her feel good—temporarily. But in digesting these "naked carbohydrates," the body has to remove vitamins (especially the B complex) and minerals from other organs to fulfill the immediate requirements for digestion and metabolism.

A food allergy can be inferred fairly definitely from a facial rash—dry, scaly cheeks, redness about the mouth, or a few pimples on forehead and chin (oily areas)—followed in a day or so by a corresponding rash (pimples) on the buttocks or a redness about the anus with cracks at the anal opening. (I can tell what holiday has just gone by—especially Easter and Halloween—by the state of the patients' buttocks.) It is psychologically difficult for the adolescent to expose his buttocks to his parents or his doctor, but if a pimple count can be made, and if the number on his face corresponds to the number on his buttocks, one should consider a food as the inciting agent. If, however, the skin of the buttocks is normal, smooth, unblemished, then perhaps the problem on the face is due merely to age and hormonal imbalance.

The usual offenders are milk (especially homogenized-pasteurized), chocolate, peanut butter (especially if hydrogenated and contaminated with additives), sugar, eggs, some cheeses (especially colored or processed), candy, and cola drinks.

If a diet change is not effective, as it should be in just a few days, assume we have arrived at Level II.

Level II for acne is pretty obvious to parents, friends, and especially to the wearer himself. Blackheads, and pimples with white heads but no real pustules, are characteristic. Most parents have been taught that this condition is the result of poor skin hygiene, and they urge scrubbing with soap and wash cloth or even a stiff brush. This acts only as a punishment, not as a therapy; it is one more stress to an already stressed skin. The blackheads are really oxidized oil, not dirt.

Assume that the skin is not functioning optimally. Up the daily intake of vitamin A to 25,000 units. Increase all the B complex to 25 to 50 mg of each of the Bs. Stop any sugar, white-flour products, and cereal, ice cream, and milk. It takes at least a month to see what a nutritional approach can do. The large intake of vitamin A is justifiable for this period of time. It may help, and I have never heard of anyone being harmed by a month on these dosages.

If this approach does not hold the adolescent skin together, then it has slipped to Level III, in which the whiteheads become infected and yellow. Pus can be expressed from these inflamed zits and the chance of permanent scarring increases. Infection suggests the use of an antibiotic, and I see no reason why anyone would want to pass up this opportunity for treatment. However, if there is improvement under this treatment, then something ought to be done to improve the patient's overall resistance to infection.

Without stopping the antibiotic, additional vitamin C, perhaps 500 to 1000 mg per day, would be appropriate. I am assuming that the advice regarding the A and B complex vitamins and no junk food is still being followed.

Here are some other things to try with Level III acne. Lecithin (three capsules three times a day) helps utilization of fatty substances, like A. Vitamin E (400 units) helps vitamin A work. Some adolescents are sensitive to iodine, so stop iodized salt and kelp for a while. Limit fish ingestion and use water-soluble vitamin A rather than fish oils. B_6, 100 mg or so per day, helps cut the oil in the skin. Slight pinkness from a sunlamp will help peel off some skin. Calcium has been helpful in some cases. Wheat germ oil or polyunsaturated salad oils should be taken daily, up to four or five teaspoons a day.

Many dermatologists have given up on the use of zinc,

but my feeling is that they have not used it simultaneously with all the other nutritional supports; 100 to 200 mg of some zinc salt added to the diet daily may show results in four to six weeks.   Many find 200 to 400 mg daily quite safe (60 to 90 mg of elemental zinc).

If the patient has moved out of Level III back to Level II, try eliminating the antibiotic for two to four weeks.   Some doctors think it works better if given intermittently, anyway. At the first sign of an infected hickey, use the maximum dose per day for three to four days.   (Some adolescents take it from Thursday to Saturday to look good on a date.)   Its long-term effects on the intestine and on the teeth and bones are not known for sure, so it should be used sparingly.

If control is attained, you or your doctor next have to decide what the combined maintenance dose of everything should be.   Change only one thing at a time, but allow no junk foods and keep up the high amounts of B and C vitamins.   Zinc is more important than vitamin A, but it probably could be reduced to 50 mg per day and finally to once a week.

If the victim also has warts, and white spots on his nails, he is more likely to respond to zinc.   If he has small bumps on the skin of his thighs and the back of his arms, he is more likely to respond to vitamin A.

Level IV acne is unsightly and disfiguring but not hope-less.   In this type, the pimples become small boils and burrow under the skin.   This disrupts the dermatological architecture so that healing produces characteristic pits and scars.   Because dermatologists have had some luck using cortisone injected directly into the cystic areas to combat inflammation, it makes some sense to help the body produce its own cortisone.   The standard diet precautions should be observed plus consumption of 100 mg of each of the B complex vitamins per day; 200 mg zinc per day; 100,000 units of vitamin A per day; vitamin C— up to 4000 to 8000 mg per day; and pantothenic acid, a B vita-min considered a cortisone precursor, 4000 to 8000 mg per day.

The contents of vitamin E capsules rubbed into the healing sores may cut down the scarring.

Try to use as many natural methods of treatment as possible. Big doses of vitamins A, B, and C and zinc may not sound "natural," but they can certainly be classified as more natural than a drug that might lead the patient to surgery. I also assume that these deficiencies in vitamins and minerals leading to skin disorders would not have occurred if the mothers had eaten the correct diet during pregnancy, if the child had eaten only natural foods during growth, and if all the foods he did eat had had all the nutrients they were supposed to have. For instance, the amount of zinc in a vegetable will vary from one area to another, depending on the amount of zinc in the topsoil where the vegetable grew. Scientists say that much zinc has been leached out of the topsoil and into the ocean, which suggests that sea salt and kelp are now better sources than spinach.

Alopecia, or hair loss, is unusual in children. Small areas of denuded skin with irregular margins could be the result of child abuse (pulling hair out in chunks), but more likely they are caused by the steady pull of a tight ponytail or rollers. Circular areas of stubble (hair about 1 to 2 mm long) are almost always the result of a fungus that gets into the hair shaft, making it brittle enough to break. A very effective antifungal agent taken orally is usually curative. However, I wonder if the presence of this condition doesn't perhaps indicate a preexisting susceptibility. When ringworm of the scalp is "going around," why don't all the children get it?

Alopecia areata (large irregular patches of denuded scalp) and alopecia totalis (all body hair falls out) are usually considered stress-related. I had a three-year-old patient who intermittently lost large swatches of hair two to three weeks after each febrile illness. I discovered that she had a kidney problem and placed her on medicine prophylactically, but her hair did not grow long and lustrous until her mother quit work and stayed home with her. I don't know what made the difference for this child. Was it the end of the separation stress? Was the diet she got at home better than the one she got at the sitter's?

A thirty-five-year-old woman told me that her total hair loss occurred six weeks after she was hit with more stress than her body could handle. In the space of two weeks her baby almost succumbed to pneumonia, her husband announced he was seeking a divorce, and both her parents died. She was able to seek medical help for the baby, legal help for the divorce, and professional handling for the funerals. But no one helped her exhausted adrenal glands. Just when she was putting her domestic and psychic life back together, out dropped her hair. A perceptive dermatologist questioned her about stress and heavy-metal poisoning (lead paint, arsenic, mercury). He gave her a cortisone product that produced a little fuzz, but he was reluctant to continue because of the known complications. She tried a nutritional approach with special emphasis on vitamin C and pantothenic acid (200 mg of each per day), and within six weeks she began to grow what appeared to be normal hair. She had had a Level V hair loss.

Why she would respond to stress with alopecia is unknown. Another person might have gotten eczema or asthma or hypertension or depression or arthritis. A disease is not as important as the mechanism that produces it. Stress produces a fall in blood sugar, the adrenals respond with cortisone and adrenalin, and if these glands are not (or were not for some time) properly nourished, the victim will be susceptible to a variety of conditions due to an insufficiency of adrenal gland hormones. The specific variant would be determined by genetic factors.

Level I hair should be lustrous, not too dry or oily and appropriate in color and texture for the particular race. If hair begins to come out in larger-than-usual amounts on comb or brush, some assessment must be made of stress factors, diet, missing nutrients, and possible toxic factors (lead, arsenic, chemical pollutants, and so on).

If the Level II hair loss can be related to stress, such as the death of a loved one, many moves, new school, disrupted family, or the like, it should be a simple matter to improve the diet and add the Stress Formula (all the B vitamins, especially pantothenic acid, and vitamin C). Hair takes a while to respond, so one must be patient for five to six weeks before doing a count of hairs taken from the brush or comb. Removing the stress, obviously, is the most important thing.

Level III is more serious; the hair loss greater and more obvious. If the therapy for stress outlined in Level II is not sufficient, it is appropriate to examine the skin and nails for other clues. White spots in the nails and warts might call for zinc—100 to 200 mg zinc gluconate for six weeks, and after that once a week. Rough skin might suggest vitamin A deficiency; give 50,000 to 100,000 units for six weeks, then cut back to once a week. Bumping into furniture in a dimly lit room also suggests that the person may not be getting enough vitamin A. (Liver, carrots and a green salad might do it overnight.)

If these clues are not manifest, a doctor's evaluation of general health and growth is in order. Chronic tonsil, gland, or kidney infection could cause physical stress sufficient to produce hair loss. A course of antibiotics or vitamin C (2000 to 6000 mg per day) should help. Anemia and lead poisoning would have to be considered. If a child is not growing according to his genetic growth potential, a number of problems come to mind. However, hair and skin defects combined with short stature suggest a zinc deficiency (*see* Autism, p. 175). There are blood tests for zinc, as well as for vitamins A and C and a few of the Bs. Some experts in nutrition consider hair analysis a more helpful method of evaluating the long-term depletion or excess of some fifteen to eighteen common and not-so-common metallic elements and poisons in our bodies.

Level IV and V hair loss means that something terrible has happened to the patient: poor diet, stress, poison, infection —probably a combination. One may need psychotherapy, standard medical therapy, medicine for mobilization and release of poisons, a rest in the country. But if the doctor says "stress" and writes out a prescription for Valium, thank him but don't fill it until the above suggestions have been tried at least twice and for at least two to three months. If he says "general exhaustion" and wants you to try cortisone, thank him for the diagnostic clue; then go home and try the Stress Formula.

Boils.   No one in Level I health ever gets a boil or any type of skin infection. A pimple or two is all right, but no boils. There is something about the integrity of healthy skin that prevents a bite, pimple, or cut from going on to become a deep, painful, throbbing, red, pus-filled boil. Usually there is a break in the skin and the dreaded staphylococcus finds this portal of entry and begins to grow. There are few other conditions in medicine that so clearly indicate how good hygiene and nutrition will preclude infection.

One boil would place the patient immediately into Level II and the chances of slipping all the way to Level V could be illustrated by a one-year-old patient of mine whose father was a chocolate-candy salesman. The boy found and ate five or six of the goodies. In three days he had a pimple (with enclosed pus) at the corner of his mouth. Somewhere he must have inhaled some of the staph germ, because in another two days he had a temperature of 105° and had turned blue from staphylococcus pneumonia. We almost lost him, and I'm sure we would have if we had used only herb tea and vitamin C when he got to that low level of resistance.

Level III is indicated by frequent pimply sores that progress to boils requiring hot packs and incision and drainage, occasionally by a surgeon. We were told about vagabonds' disease in medical school. It is an illness usually suffered only by the unwashed and ill-fed; occasionally a clean, well-fed but apparently not well-nourished patient will get this chronic skin infection.

A patient in my recent memory was helped by the use of 50,000 units of vitamin A daily (because A helps the skin maintain itself and she had that characteristic bumpy texture on the back of her upper arms indicative of vitamin A deficiency), zinc gluconate (50 mg daily), and 1000 mg of vitamin C (it seems to enhance resistance to infection), in addition to the elimination of chocolate, cola drinks, sugar, and white flour. A potent B complex also was added. In a month the boil count was down by half and in six months boils appeared only rarely and disappeared rapidly. Her problem was another illustration of the fact that we are all different. Her diet and daily habits were no different from those of others without her condition, but she had a genetic need to be supernourished in vitamins A and C and zinc.

If she had slipped to Level IV, a more thorough workup would have been called for, to include allergy testing (a milk allergy can allow this susceptibility); blood studies for anemia, white blood-cell function, and level of gamma globulin (the body's circulating immunity factor); and perhaps a hair analysis (to discover some hidden mineral imbalance).

Some doctors have had luck using a vaccine made of the patient's own staphylococcus. In this treatment, a solution of the germs (killed, of course) is injected back into the patient at weekly intervals. This will sometimes immunize him against the staph germs. Sometimes a stock vaccine will work as well. Antibiotics daily have little prophylactic use.

This tough and ubiquitous germ is on everyone's skin

and nose and throat membranes, and when stress occurs, or the body's fantastic immune system turns its back for a second, the germ sneaks in and lodges in a joint (septic arthritis), a bone (osteomyelitis), a kidney (abscess), the brain (meningitis), or a lung (staphylococcal pneumonia). If a patient finds himself with any of these severe, destructive, sometimes overwhelming infections, he obviously needs the full attention and therapeutic support of the doctor in the hospital, because he is at the bottom Level V. While he is surviving—if he survives—he should be receiving, along with heroic doses of anti-staphylococcal antibiotics, massive doses of vitamin C (maybe 1000 mg intravenously every hour for a day or so), and a lot of B complex vitamins. Few other diseases distress the body as much as the invasion of this nasty germ. When the germs are dead and the patient is home, some effort must be made to figure out what is wrong with his genes, his diet, or his lifestyle.

Bites from insects are experienced by most of us. I imagine even a Level I person might occasionally serve as a target for an angry bee or wasp or provide a meal for a hungry mosquito, flea, or gnat. But nutritionists seem to believe that bugs will not bother someone who is optimally nourished, perhaps because the skin is so tough they cannot penetrate it. I remember, while on a fishing trip, watching a mosquito land on my hand. It sniffed around and flew away, apparently nauseated from the smell of the brewer's yeast that was oozing through my pores. It is quite possible that variables in the individual may preclude the consistent benefits of brewer's yeast, but try it. If it works, use it. It is water-soluble, so it must be taken every two to four hours. Insect repellent may work better. Cortisone ointment will calm the itch, as will vitamin E oil.

The Level II or Level III person hates being bitten because he is a histamine releaser. He is an allergic person and a flea bite is a major trauma. He usually is more likely than the Level I person to get hives and have dermatographia. He should follow the Basic Diet plus the Stress Formula to alleviate his misery, but if he has to scratch, he will be susceptible to impetigo or boils.

The Level IV person is the one who overreacts to bee stings. Adolescent males seem to be the most susceptible. If someone collapses within ten to twenty minutes after the sting of a bee, hornet, yellowjacket, or wasp with fainting, shock, hives, or asthma, he is in Level V and needs emergency treatment—adrenalin, oxygen, and possibly cortisone. He needs to carry the bee-sting emergency kit at all times and should also be desensitized to the venom. Some authorities feel that the only acceptable vaccine is the extracted venom. Until a better answer is found, assume that the victim has troubled adrenal glands and that he should follow the Basic Diet plus the Stress Formula, with additional intake of pantothenic acid and vitamin C—even increasing the intake of the latter two vitamins up to 3000 mg per day prior to entering an area of a possible sting. (Don't forget the kit!)

If you would prefer to treat bee stings naturally, use fresh cow manure. The freshness is what counts, so be prepared to follow the cow around with a sheet. When you have accumulated plenty of manure, wrap the sheet with its contents about the sting area of the victim and leave it on all night. In the morning all evidence of the sting will be gone.

Burns are terribly painful and constitute a major stress for the body. A Level I burn would be a slight pinkness after some exposure to the sun; in two days it turns to a beautiful coppery tan. We all should be so lucky!

Level II could be caused by scalding soup or coffee spilled on a hand or on the chest, but involving an area no bigger than five inches square. Before and instead of rushing off to the emergency room or plastering it with butter or lard, immerse the hand in ice water—not cold water, *ice* water—and keep it there for two to four hours—not minutes, *hours.* A burn on the chest or any other area that cannot be immersed should be covered with a wet cloth and kept wet with ice cubes for the same length of time. Research indicates that this emergency treatment will keep a first-degree burn from becoming a second-degree burn and a second-degree burn from becoming third-degree.

Whether or not a victim is taken to the doctor later for evaluation and possible bandaging, the ice is always the first thing. Vitamin E capsules can be opened and the oil squeezed onto the burn. This is safe, kills the pain, and in the opinion of some promotes healing with little scarring. I would not object to aspirin or even codeine to ease the suffering. Add the Stress Formula as soon as possible. All can be used simultaneously.

An extensive fire burn would drop the patient into Level V and, of course, into medical and surgical management. It seems absurd to see a burn patient being managed with all the modern facilities of aseptic care, with blood and plasma given intravenously, with the most scientific ointments and surgery prescribed, but with no extra nutritional supports for the skin and adrenal glands. At no other time in the life of the patient will his body need supernutrition more than when he is burned severely. He should have 1000 mg of vitamin C every hour for the first few days, along with 200 to 500 mg of all the B vitamins. Vitamin A, up to 100,000 units a day for a few days, and 90 mg of elemental zinc for maybe two to four weeks, should be near the top of the list. If you are a relative of a burn victim, insist that these nutrients be included. Some doctors think they will be considered quacks if they order them, but they can be reassured that the information has been tested repeatedly and found effective. The extra zinc—even if you have to smuggle it into the hospital—has been shown to cut healing time in half. If you are in charge or in attendance when the dressings are changed, that's the time to apply the vitamin E oil from the capsules to cut down scarring .

Candidiasis is the fairly common yeast infection that seems to bedevil bottle-fed babies, especially those from mothers who have a vaginal yeast infection. It is more likely to appear when there is a vitamin A deficiency. It usually follows the taking of an antibiotic; the normal bacteria are suppressed, allowing for the growth of this ubiquitous yeast.

A Level I baby would be breast-fed and would have come from a mother who did not have the infection; the baby would, of course, be free of rashes.

In Level II, the baby might show some white spots on his gums or inside his cheeks. They look like milk curds, but they don't come off without causing bleeding. This condition is called thrush. It might go away by itself, but using vitamin C (100 mg per day for the baby and 1000 mg per day for the mother), boroglycerin on a swab, zephiran hydrochloride suitably diluted, and nature's own acidophyllus bifidus bacteria all will make them go away faster.

If thrush is accompanied by a very red, solid rash in the diaper area with a sharp line of small blisters where it borders normal skin, it becomes more serious and an antiyeast medicine (Nystatin) would be appropriate. However, this condition surely indicates that Level III or IV has been reached and that both mother and baby should be placed in the risk category. The Stress Formula plus the Prevention Diet for the mother (she should have been on it anyway, since she was recently pregnant) should be started and the baby given maybe 200 mg of vitamin C per day for a few days, plus up to 25 mg of each of the Bs, plus 10,000 to 20,000 mg of vitamin A, plus the acidophyllus. The Nystatin is given orally and also used in a cream.

Cuts are common in children, probably because they have skin and frequently don't watch what they are doing. A Level 1 child might never get cut all his life. Most cuts longer than an inch call for a doctor's evaluation as to the need for suturing. But a doctor will generally suture as a matter of course, so for minor cuts it will be worthwhile to consider the following:

1. A scar will form in size comparable to the gape of the fresh wound, so you must decide if you can live with the size and location of that particular scar. When the bleeding stops and you have washed it for several minutes with fresh water, pat it dry and pinch the wound edges together. If the edges fit neatly, tape them together with butterfly or paper closure tapes. If scared or nervous, call the doctor.

2. If a wound has not closed in eight to twelve hours, it probably should be left open, since infection might prevent proper healing.

3. If the taping method has achieved a thin line of closure, you probably don't need the surgeon. Wounds on knees and elbows, however, always need suturing, since the elastic tissue can't be held by tapes. Tapes are best for the half-inch cuts of the forehead and chin of the one- to three-year-old who is absolutely petrified by the scary emergency room.

Rub a little vitamin E oil on the healing wound daily. The better the blood supply, the more rapid the healing process: face and head, three to four days; arms and trunk, seven to ten days; legs and feet, ten days to two weeks. If the cut gets more red and tender after three days, it is getting infected. It means you did not wash the wound thoroughly with running water before you closed it, or there is dirt or foreign matter still in the wound, or you forgot the vitamin C—1000 to 2000 mg per day during healing. Swallow your pride and call the doctor.

Superficial crustiness can be treated with an antibiotic ointment such as Polymycin or Neomycin, which will kill some germs (*see* Impetigo, later in this chapter).

Any wounds that penetrate beneath the skin into muscle, bone, tendon, or into the abdomen, or which involve the eye, ear, nose, or an exposed tooth, are in the III, IV, or V category, and the surgeon is required. Don't fool around.

A child who cuts or burns himself frequently is accident-prone. Consider what can be done to help him better perceive where he is in space.

Dermatographia is the phenomenon of easy and rapid production of wheals or welts on the skin when lightly stroked with almost any object. You can write your name or play tic-tac-toe on the skin of such a person. The pressure disturbs white cells that release histamine. The histamine makes local blood vessels swell and ooze serum, producing redness with central pallor. Because cortisone inhibits this response, the dermatographic person may be allergic. He probably has some symptoms (hay fever, stomachaches, headaches, phlegm, possibly asthma) that could be alleviated by taking the Stress Formula with extra vitamin C (1000 mg per day) and by changes in the diet.

With Level II people, it takes a lot of firm pressure to leave a red line on the skin and that disappears quickly. This person probably sneezes some and has gas with some foods, but he is in no big trouble. Maybe just using the Prevention Diet and vitamins and eliminating aggravating foods, pets, and pollens is enough.

Level III and IV people with very reactive skin should

make some effort to move out of these levels, since their bodies are at risk for allergic problems. The more the skin is responsive to touch, the more pantothenic acid (a cortisone precursor) is required, even up to 1000 to 5000 mg per day until the dermatographia is reduced.

Dandruff often runs in families, suggesting an inherited tendency or a family allergy to milk. But it may also mean a deficiency of B vitamins in the diet of each family member. Cradle cap might be the first clue that the baby will have a lifelong problem. If a mother had nausea and vomiting during the pregnancy (usually a B_6 deficiency) and if her new baby has cradle cap (dandruff or seborrhea), she knows that the baby needs extra B_6 (it is best to give all the Bs), 20 to 50 mg per day for a while for both of them.

Skin-loosening shampoos are helpful, but there is a reason that the flaky skin and scales keep coming back. A month of 50,000 to 100,000 units of vitamin A for the six-year-old to adult might tell something. Zinc may be a factor. Not enough linoleic acid can do the same thing. Some find that vitamin E (400 to 1200 units) taken internally and as an ointment calms down the showers of skin (E makes A work better). See Chapter 2 for foods rich in these vitamins and minerals.

If an adolescent has dandruff with his acne, all his skin might clear up with B_6, 100 mg; vitamin A, 50,000 units; linoleic acid and zinc, 100 mg per day.

Hair is composed mainly of protein, but it requires minerals and B vitamins to become lustrous and manageable. If the Prevention Diet and vitamins have little effect, vitamin A, 50,000 to 100,000 units for five to six weeks, might improve the texture. Zinc might be tried next, since it catalyzes the enzyme that lays down protein in the skin and probably in the hair.

In many cases, gray hair has been returned to its original color with the Prevention Diet plus vitamins, but with special emphasis on whole grains; brewer's yeast; PABA (para amino-benzoic acid), 200 to 300 mg per day; and pantothenic acid, 100 mg or more per day. All are very safe.

Eczema is the "itch that rashes." It is a giveaway that the victim will have allergic problems all his life. It is assumed to be familial and is made worse with stress and poor diet. Cortisone by mouth and injection will control most cases, but one of the ideas of nutritional health is to try to avoid powerful hormones. The side effects and the danger of getting "hooked" are an unfortunate tradeoff to the great and immediate benefits of its use. Usually when a synthetic hormone is introduced into the body, its passage through the blood vessels of the pituitary causes that gland to secrete less of its stimulating hormone (in this case ACTH, adrenocorticotrophic hormone) so that the target gland (in this case, the adrenal cortex) will secrete less. Thus, if cortisone is given, the adrenal cortex will produce less. When the patient and the doctor decide the eczema is better and the shots or pills are discontinued, the eczema will flare up more viciously than ever because the adrenal glands have not had a chance to tool up; or the patient was not nourishing his adrenal glands sufficiently for them to take over.

It is interesting to note that few breast-fed babies develop eczema. In bottle-fed babies the rash appears two to six weeks after birth, which would suggest that the protective hormones from the mother had finally washed out of the baby and his adrenal glands were not producing enough cortisone to save him from this mess.

But there is never simply one factor in eczema. Also contributing in some degree are familial or genetic tendencies, ingestion of cow's milk, improper nourishment or stress during the pregnancy, and a difficult delivery. Zinc also seems to be a factor in eczema. The zinc in cow's milk (if the cow has been eating enough fodder that contains zinc) may be bound up with protein, and some humans cannot digest protein well enough to get the zinc out of it.

A Level II eczema shows as circular red scaly patches on the cheeks. The child might try to dig at them or rub his face on the sheets. The doctor will supply you with a free sample of cortisone ointment as a diagnostic test; rub it sparingly on one spot only two or three times a day. In twenty-four hours the treated area should be almost clear compared to the untreated one. If so, one is assured that it is the start of eczema (or some related allergy), and immediate steps should be taken to build up the child's adrenal glands. (1) Don't give up nursing; or, if you already have, go back to it if it is not too late. (2) If you are nursing, stop your ingestion of dairy products, chocolate, wheat, eggs, citrus foods, and tomato. (3) Stop giving the baby any vitamin drops that have coloring, sugar, flavoring, or additives. (4) Begin some vitamin C (100 mg per day at first, larger doses if nothing happens) and pantothenic acid (100 mg at first per day, perhaps double or triple this in a few days if there are no results). Grind up the tablets in water; smile as you poke this down.

If nothing happens in a few days, or if the eczema gets worse, you have made the wrong diagnosis (*see* Candidiasis, above), or your baby cannot absorb these nutriments fast enough (maybe he should have a shot of vitamin B complex with pantothenic acid), or he has slipped into Level III.

In this level he becomes miserable; the rash has spread to most of his face, scalp, and ears and shows up in the front of his elbows and the back of his knees. If he is bottle-fed, he should be changed to soybean milk. In three days he should be less irritable and the rash less angry-looking. (Try to find a milk without sucrose, dextrose, or corn syrup.)

Before the baby slips into a level where the doctor might suggest cortisone, add a chelated zinc to the diet, at least 50 mg a day. Zinc is thought to be essential to the enzyme that allows RNA synthesis of skin protein; with less than an optimum amount the skin cannot repair itself properly.

Before cortisone is used internally (or even suggested), try to find a doctor who will prescribe some of the ointments used in the precortisone era (coal-tar derivatives), or use a locally applied cortisone cream that has the lowest percentage of cortisone. I have been amazed at how quickly many of these babies clear up and become more comfortable with a vitamin B complex injection. Maybe the B vitamins help the adrenal glands, but maybe the B vitamins help the intestinal enzymes function better to digest and absorb the fat and zinc.

Soap, of course, is taboo with eczema. Cleanse with oil and use only soft cotton next to the skin. Benadryl is a safe antihistamine that will have a quieting effect on the skin and a calming effect on the baby, but many find different herb teas work as well and that dolomite powder (up to 1000 mg of calcium, 500 mg of magnesium) is a safe calming agent. Because skin is involved, at least 10,000 and up to 50,000 units of vitamin A would be worthwhile. Alternating milk—from raw cow's milk to goat's to soy, to lamb-base, to an amino-acid milk—may be helpful. Some have found that when allergies are rampant in the family and the mother is unable to nurse the baby, eczema can be avoided by beginning on day one with soy milk. Try vitamin E oil to soften the skin.

Eczema patients frequently have trouble with absorption of oil-soluble vitamins and consequently with linoleic acid, an essential fatty acid for the integrity of the skin. Cod-liver oil is best for vitamins A and D (enough to supply 25,000 units of A and 1000 units of D for a month), plus a teaspoon a day of some vegetable oil containing linoleic acid.

Patients outgrow much of this condition in time but they remain susceptible to its recurrence or to some such other allergic problem as intestinal allergies or asthma. These peo-

ple, more than anyone else, have to stick to the Prevention
Diet and the Stress Formula with vitamins and zinc for their
lifetimes.

Take note, however: the doses mentioned above are
approximations for the two- to ten-month-old. Older children
and adults might require more, but these are good values to
start with. Try one thing at a time and stay with each approach for at least three or four weeks before altering or drop-
ping it. (In general, large doses of vitamins A and D and the
minerals should be reduced after one to two months to those
recommended in Chapter 2; vitamins B and C can be continued in mega amounts.)

Fungus conditions are now felt to be the failure of an
unhealthy skin to cleanse itself of a parasite lying on its surface. They are usually recognized by the owner, the mother,
or the school coach as athlete's foot, jock-strap itch, or ringworm of the skin. Some over-the-counter creams and pow-
ders containing undecylenic acid are beneficial.

If one has fungus, one treats it, but it is also a clue that
the body has slipped to a level where more than just local
treatment is called for. The diet must be changed and the
basic vitamin and mineral formula added.

If it continues or recurs (Level III), a doctor's attention
is needed. He can prescribe a very effective medicine. The
special skin formula below must be followed, and prehaps a
soap change is worthwhile.

Six-year-old to adolescent daily: increase cod-liver oil to
1000 units of D, 25,000 units of A; 100 mg zinc (especially if
white spots are noted in nails); one tablespoon of some vegetable oil (soy, safflower, sunflower, or the like): one or two
pancreatic granules with each meal: vitamin C, quadruple
what is now being taken. Do all this for four to six weeks,
then settle back to a maintenance dose. White spots in the

nails, flaking skin, tiny bumps on the back of the arms, and cheesy smell to the socks might indicate that one is in or about to be in trouble again.

Level IV fungus problems need the dermatologist's attention. Fungus is in the hair shafts or is eating away at the nails. An internal fungicide (Griseofulvin) is usually curative, but the therapy in the preceding paragraph would make it more efficiently curative and, of course, would cheer the dermatologist.

Ichthyosis is the fish skin that some people inherit. Vitamin A, especially the water-soluble kind (25,000 to 50,000 units), may help in some of these cases. Vitamin E helps A work better and also might be applied locally.

Impetigo, like skin fungus, is a clue that something has happened to the skin to allow an invasion of the normal skin population, in this case streptococcus or staphylococcus. The usual story is that the child has skinned his knee, elbow, or chin and has then breathed on the wound and picked at the scab. Instead of healing, the area becomes tender and red, and yellow pus oozes from the edges of the crust. Redness spreads to adjacent skin, and occasionally red streaks (lymphangitis) will form as the poison advances.

Level I people do not get this following a cut or abrasion because of good resistance. Level II people have only to add the Stress Formula for a few days, plus zinc (up to 100 mg per day for ten days), plus rubbing on vitamin E oil alternately with some over-the-counter antibiotic cream, plus bathing and use of large sterile pads to splint the skin.

If Level III has been reached (with spreading infection, oozing pus, and swollen lymph nodes near the area) a doctor's help is the wisest course, because the dreaded glomerulonephritis (kidney disease) can follow some innocuous-looking scabby sore. The doctor is supposed to prescribe penicillin or erythromycin for ten days to prevent a plunge to Level IV. Obviously, something has made the body highly susceptible. While one is wondering, 1000 mg of vitamin C five to ten times a day would be helpful. (The suggestions for control of skin stress should be followed; *see* Fungus, above.)

Nails on the fingers and toes give important clues as to general state of recent health, richness of diet, and levels of some minerals and vitamins. The nails give this information, just as the annular rings of a tree chronicle its good and bad years.

Thin and weak nails suggest a chronic disease or low-protein diet. Pale nails suggest low iron or at least anemia. Blue nails mean poorly oxygenated blood or a circulatory, lung, or heart problem. White spots represent healed injuries, but spots numbering more than a few may indicate a clue to a zinc deficiency. Fine linear ridges may be a specific protein or B complex insufficiency; some feel a B_6 lack is the cause.

Nails need protein that is rich in sulfur-containing amino acids (as in eggs). High doses of B vitamins, as in brewer's yeast and sunflower seeds, are good for nails. Calcium will toughen them. Choline too—500 to 1500 mg per day—is a good nail-builder.

Perspiration, when excessive, is the response some people have to stress. It is a clue that the body is disturbed about something. The mind says the situation is "really nothing," but here are the drippy hands, feet, and armpits that betray the anxiety. The embarrassment caused by the moisture in social situations is stress enough to cause further perspiration, until the victim can bear it no longer and avoids what could be fun activities.

The meaning of the excess sweating, like heart palpitations, feelings of impending doom, crying jags, shyness, and so on, can be looked for in the etiology of the great group of stress-caused illnesses. These moist people perceive stress in their brain while there may be no palpable stress in the environment.

Doctors have powerful medicines to cut the perception of stress (at Level IV), but some attention should be paid to the limbic system (*see* Chapter 9) to raise its threshold of awareness. Hypoglycemia may play a role, and the Prevention Diet and vitamin program may be helpful.

Psychiatric intervention may be necessary after the above suggestions are tried. Surgical intervention—cutting the nerves that stimulate sweat glands—must be considered a Level V approach; it would be unfortunate to go through surgery and then find you were still sweating from an unresolved Oedipus complex.

Pityriasis alba is characterized by a white, scaly, circular patch usually on the cheeks of children who have a mild food allergy, usually to milk. The condition is fairly common and not serious. The white circles are more noticeable at the end of summer because they do not tan after exposure to the sun.

Because they do clear up by themselves in a couple of years, and because they don't itch or get infected, they usually are ignored once diagnosed. The reason they are even mentioned in this book is to indicate that the bearer has fallen from Level I. Because a cortisone salve will make these areas recede faster than time alone, it suggests that the adrenals are on the weak side and that if hay fever, gas, ear infections, circles under the eyes, or dermatographia are not already present, one or more of these conditions could soon appear and drag the Level II victim into deeper trouble.

This is just a clue, mind you, but that is what this book is about: helping you figure out where the tilt is before you fall over into a diagnosable disease category.

Obviously, stop the milk, add the vitamins and minerals, follow the Prevention Diet and the adrenal gland and skin support programs and wait until next summer. If the skin's tan is even, not patchy-looking, you have done it, but if everything is worse, repeat these programs but in bigger doses.

Poison oak, poison ivy, and *contact dermatitis* in general are short-lived, albeit miserable, problems. Some people can dive into toxic greenery and suffer not at all: these have to be Level I people (at least for this). They are often the people, justifiably proud, who say "Mind over matter."

Here again, if someone gets a skin rash from plants, paint, plastic, toilet seats, cosmetics, belts, nylon shoes (the list is endless), he or she is allergic. The level of the problem is determined by how miserable they are—itch, extent of rash, amount of insomnia, and so forth. If one knows he has been exposed to something he is sensitive to, especially poison oak, he should thoroughly cleanse the skin with soap and water as soon after exposure as possible and wash the clothes that are contaminated. These measures may prevent a rash from appearing. When the poison oak or ivy rash begins, it gets worse for five days, then better for five days. The sufferer can speed recovery by taking big doses of vitamin C (1000 mg every one to three hours), one to two grams of dolomite (calcium cuts pain and magnesium inhibits the histamine release), and all the B vitamins, especially pantothenic acid (500 to 3000 mg per day).

Cortisone has been a sanity-saver for people in Level IV or V, but the need for it suggests that the adrenals must be nourished. To avoid future bouts, the Prevention Diet and the

Stress Formula should be followed. Then, after three to four months, stick your little finger in a poison oak leaf and see if you are in better shape adrenally. If unsure, keep the vitamin A under 50,000 units per day after six weeks.

Prickly heat is an extensive rash that prickles and itches and is concentrated where there are sweat glands. It comes from a combination of high external heat, clothing that chafes, and some unknown stress factor. Some parents overdress their new baby so he won't get a chill—but he may get prickly heat and a fever.

Vitamin C seems to stop it overnight. Dosages are infants, 100 to 200 mg per day; children, 250 to 1000 mg per day; and adults, 1000 to 3000 mg per day. Two to four days should be enough. Also, exposing the skin to circulating air seems sensible.

The appearance of prickly heat suggests a stressful reaction to climate, but it can be a clue that other sicknesses or stress-related conditions are lurking. Follow the Prevention Diet and continue the vitamin program indefinitely, and be ready to pump in extra vitamin C at any sneeze, itch, irritability, or weather change.

Psoriasis is not seen much in children—or perhaps pediatricians are unable to recognize its early manifestations. It is usually diagnosed by excluding other similar conditions. Its cause is a combination of genetic, stress and nutritional factors. It may show up suddenly like a contagious disease, or it may break out slowly area by area. It is more likely to occur in the extensor areas of the knees, elbows, wrists, scalp, buttocks, and back. When it settles in as chronic, it is a reddened base with a thin, scaly, tissue-paper surface.

A dermatologist is required who may have to try a number of things, so don't assume he is not knowledgable. He is trying to find the treatment that is best for you and your skin. (Oral medicine plus ultraviolet light is the current favorite.)

His treatments will control the condition better if you are using the Prevention Diet and the Stress Formula. (If you didn't have stress at the onset, you have it once you know the diagnosis.) The vitamins for skin nutrition are: vitamin A, 25,000 to 100,000 units per day for six weeks, depending on age; zinc, 60 to 90 mg per day for six weeks, depending on age; vegetable oils; pancreatic enzymes at each meal (maybe absorption of something essential is off); lecithin, three capsules three times a day for about six weeks.

What you are trying to forestall is the doctor's use of cortisone and/or methoxsalen, which is a drug that slows cell growth (it might slow up some other cells you need).

Scabies is the seven-year itch caused by a very hungry, pregnant little insect that burrows just under the skin surface (like a garden mole), laying her eggs as she goes. The presence of these parasites and eggs causes an intense itching, and the resulting scratching and infection sometimes make the diagnosis difficult.

Some health authorities feel that healthy skin, like a healthy garden, will not attract ticks, lice, chiggers, fungi, but I am not so sure. If we are full of the proper nutrients, wouldn't we make a better feast? (Bugs avoid white bread.) Nevertheless, healthy, tough skin is hard to burrow into.

Scabies lesions usually are linear and in warm, thin areas—pulse side of wrist, front fold of armpit, warm parts of groin, webs of fingers.

Improve the diet and add the stress and skin program so infection won't follow, but also apply some benzyl benzoate

(Kwell). The nutritional approach alone may take seven years.

Sunburn is a stress and should be treated with the Stress Formula as soon as possible. PABA, 1000 mg, and vitamin E, 400 units, can promote healing. Calcium dulls the pain. Better to use the PABA on the skin before the exposure; it is the operative ingredient in sunscreen lotions. Nothing else works as well, except keeping fully clothed. Vitamin A (25,000 units per day) and calcium carbonate (120 mg per day) may protect the fair skinned.

Varicose veins are now routinely treated with vitamin E, 800 to 1200 units per day. Vitamin C, 500 to 1000 mg per day, will make the damaged tissues pull together. Bioflavenoids enhance the vitamin C here. This is, of course, in addition to the Prevention Diet.

Many observers feel that constipation and straining to get a big bowel movement out causes or at least contributes to varicosities, especially on the upper left thigh. These veins have to drain upward into the pelvis, and if a large stool is sitting there (the colon is on the left side), it will create a hydrostatic pressure and stretch the veins in the legs. One must avoid constipating foods and tight girdles or binding garments.

Warts have been treated with everything, because everything works on warts. The idea is to do something, *anything*, that you believe in and they will dry up and fall off. The point is that warts are a clue that the skin has lost its ability to keep the wart virus from invading.

Vitamin A, 100,000 units per day, and zinc, 60 mg per day, for four to six weeks is the standard nutritional attack on warts, assuming one is following the Prevention Diet. Knowing how the mind can affect the body, I am not surprised that hypnosis can achieve almost identical results. There is a limit, however, and the hypnotically treated patient is more likely to suffer a recurrence when the body runs out of the means to control the situation. □

Can you write your name on your child's skin with your fingernail? That red line is supposed to be due to a histamine release. It is a clue that he is allergy prone. Throw down some extra pantothenic acid (200 to 500 mg per day) and try again.

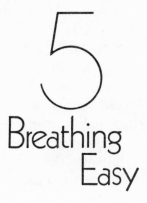

Breathing Easy

Respiratory infections and respiratory allergies are the most common reasons for phone calls and visits to the doctor. The impression we got as medical students was that every child gets sick with a cold, cough, influenza, sore throat, and accompanying complications about four to six times a year. At greater frequencies, an allergy would be suspected.

The notion that children (and adults) who often have colds, coughs, or sore throats are inadequately nourished was never seriously considered, since malnutrition occurs mainly in poor or underdeveloped countries. Yet some of our children are not sick at all, some are sick an average amount, and some are sick all the time. Could some of the more sickly ones be malnourished? If we find out what the parents are doing for the well ones and apply it to the sick ones, can we change these averages? Up to now, we have only been able to say "A lot of babies get colds" or "It's probably an allergy."

Our Level I child never gets a cold, maybe sneezes once or twice a month, and only coughs if exposed to overwhelming

71

pollution or if milk runs down his windpipe. The child is usually breast-fed. His mother had a stressless pregnancy with no nausea and vomiting, his delivery was full-term and "normal," and he was pink and breathed well. No stress.

The children I see who have frequent colds (often accompanied by ear infections) often come from parents who have allergies. Usually the mother was not quite adequately nourished because she suffered in pregnancy from nausea and vomiting or from a threatened miscarriage, high blood pressure, or toxemia. Or, she says, she just felt uncomfortable, tired, or irritable. Her obstetrician may have prevented her from gaining more than twenty pounds for the nine months. She may have delivered the child prematurely. As a consequence of one or more of these factors, coupled with a difficult delivery, the child has suffered stress.

It is interesting that these babies seem to be comfortable until age three to five weeks, when they fall apart with some "psychosomatic" problem: colic, eczema, asthma, hay fever, diarrhea. The target area in the body appears to be determined by genetic forces; someone in the family has (or had) a similar weakness in the intestinal, respiratory, or skin department. In general, then, allergy problems show up in babies who have suffered a stress severe enough to "exhaust" their adrenal glands. The three-to-five-week latent period from delivery to illness is just about the right amount of time for the adrenals to run out of the hormones that protect the victim from the onslaught of his allergy. (Lots of babies suffer stress and don't succumb by showing some "disease." This final step into sickness is probably a result of some genetic predisposition.)

It is not too far-fetched to assume that the mother's body provided the baby with enough supportive hormones before birth to give him passive protection until the three to five weeks passed. It could also be assumed that the pregnancy stress had a debilitating effect on the mother's adrenals and that the baby's adrenals might have been called upon to help her out before birth; then, at birth, if nothing was done to revitalize the baby's adrenals, he would slip into an allergic situation that would provide a continuation of the stress that got him into the metabolic hole in the first place. A vicious cycle: stress causes more stress.

The final stroke to this dismal picture comes when the mother—reinforced by worried friends and relatives and her obstetrician—is urged to go to the bottle. They assume that the stress of nursing will exhaust her even more, which may or may not be true. So the very baby who should not be given cow's milk because of its allergenic tendencies is the one who gets it.

Every effort should be made to nurse this stress-prone child to prevent him from slipping into an uncomfortable level. When the mother is unable to nurse, she has the option of using a wet nurse or contacting the La Leche League (*see* Bibliography and Additional Helps, p. 243) to obtain human milk. Nursing for even a few days might give the baby enough of the early milk (colostrum) to get his immune and anti-allergic systems operating.

I believe that any mother who finds herself at the end of her pregnancy with any of the above conditions and who knows a little of the family's genetic susceptibility to allergies should—nay, must—fortify herself and her baby with extra amounts of the Stress Formula or insist on a few B complex and C injections from her doctor. She also should rise above the negative counsel of family and professionals and nurse her baby. She would be wise to give her baby extra vitamin C and B complex in the first few weeks of its life (*see* Anti-Infection Program, chapter 3). Prevention is always a better treatment than waiting for the disease to become manifest.

Asthma is the noisy breathing that results from the passage of air through the narrowed bronchial tubes. It is considered a severe form of respiratory allergy, sometimes appearing *de novo* and sometimes as the end stage of hay fever, postnasal drip, or months of snorting, zonking, and nocturnal dry cough. I consider it serious enough to place the victim in a Level IV category; if blueness and severe anxiety accompany the wheeze, the child is Level V and usually requires hospitalization.

When someone—child or adult—is asthmatic, a doctor is usually necessary to bail him out. He may do a test series for allergy, possibly calling for skin tests, antiwheeze medicines, and a dust-free environment. All this is standard, and the directions should be followed to the letter. But one might balk when cortisone (orally or by injections) is suggested; it certainly does help and may be almost life-saving, but side effects such as impaired growth, compromised immune systems, diabetes, and stomach ulcers may be the price.

If one has time (the child can eat, breathe, and sleep) and the asthma is partially controlled with ephedrine, aminophylline, and other antiwheeze medicines, a heroic attempt should be made to pull the adrenals back together. A good general rule is this: if cortisone will help a condition, the body with the condition has weakened adrenals, due either to stress or failure of the diet to provide enough of the adrenal hormone precursors. These are, in general, vitamin C, vitamin B_6, pantothenic acid, and vitamin A. Actually, *all* the vitamins, minerals, and amino acids are required, but these four seem to be most important.

Not everyone will respond to the above, so some experimenting has to be done. Vitamin E may be important, since it helps make vitamin A work more efficiently and is worthwhile if pollution is a prominent factor. Vitamin B_{12} has been known to eliminate asthma in some people. Calcium can relax the muscles surrounding the bronchial tubes; it also alters the permeability of the cell walls, allowing the nutrients to get it. We have seen some patients take big doses of the above with no results until a mixed B complex and vitamin C injection is given; the problem is then believed to be inefficient intestinal absorption. (Intravenous vitamin C, five grams, and calcium gluconate, one gram, may stop an asthma attack.)

Allergy Program

The suggested dosages that follow are taken for three to four weeks, beginning with lower dosages at one to three weeks of age and reaching maximum at ages ten years to adulthood.

- Vitamin A, 100,000 units daily; cut back after a month
- Vitamin C, 200 mg daily to 10,000 mg daily
- Vitamin B complex, 50 to 200 mg daily
- Pantothenic acid, 100 to 4000 mg daily
- Vitamin E, 50 units to 1200 units daily
- Vitamin B_{12}, 50 micrograms to 1 mg (probably best intramuscularly) daily
- Calcium, at least 1000 mg, should be given daily. Vitamin D (400 to 1000 units) will promote utilization.

Hypoglycemia (or any stress) can affect the adrenal glands, so it is advisable that the treatment program include the nibbling, six-meals-per-day protein diet.

If some control is achieved, the doses might be cut back to near or slightly above the recommended doses for chronic stress; these doses may have to be continued for a lifetime. One can never achieve Level I health with a family history of allergies or the pregnancy stresses, but one might be able to stay at Level II or III.

If these nutritional suggestions are not helpful, an exercise program, transcendental meditation, reflexology, biofeedback, acupuncture, and hypnosis might be helpful. Chiropractors have been known to work wonders in many cases.   A move to Arizona gets a patient away from the doctor who has run out of ideas, and it may even solve the wheeze if the problem was caused by a moldy basement or ragweed. Most people who move, however, find that they have to take their worn-out adrenals with them and the tight chest soon returns.

Bad breath may be caused by almost any dysfunction from the lips to the anus, from the sinuses to the liver. Infections of the nose, throat, gums, lungs, and intestines are reasonably obvious sources. Children frequently shove available minutia into available orifices and then forget about them. Nothing smells worse than the odor coming from a child's nostril a week or so after he has pushed a button, bean, or bit of tissue up his nose. A frontal attack is usually futile, since it is more likely to push the object farther up the tunnel. Before seeking professional help, an enterprising parent might try to force the object out by blowing into the child's mouth. The air curves around the palate and pushes the infected mess out. A child who puts things in his nose usually has a nasal allergy; he is trying to scratch the mucosa inside.

When the breath is foul, tonsils should not be removed merely because they are enlarged. Infected postnasal drip may be the cause of the odor and of the irritated tonsils. Another possible cause of bad breath is milk; try eliminating it for a month and then sniff around. People who eat animal protein (especially beef) are likely to have bad breath and pass foul-smelling gas because of the action of putrefactive bacteria. The obnoxious products are absorbed and somehow escape the cleansing action of the liver. They pass via the blood to the lungs, where they are exhaled. Changing the diet and taking some digestive enzymes may be helpful.

Bloody noses, or *epistasis,* in children and adults are frequent for many reasons. In winter, dry air dries out the nasal membranes, which crack and bleed. In cases of nasal allergy,

the blood supply to the nose is increased, and frequent blowing and sneezing may break a vessel. Some people seem to be
genetically prone to bleed from an area just inside on the septum; a little oil or petroleum jelly may help keep the area soft
and pliable.

I was a frequent victim of blood dripping from my
nose, and in spite of a variety of treatments, including cauteri-
zation with silver nitrate and hot needles, it continued until I
increased my vitamin C intake to 500 mg per day. I had nasal
scurvy for ten years.

One of my patients had nocturnal nosebleeds. I thought
gravity had something to do with it, and told his mother to sit
up all night and watch him. About 2 A.M. he began to pick his
nose in his sleep. The itch that made him scratch was due to
the fuzzy panda bear he slept with. The bleeding stopped
the night he got a bear stuffed with foam rubber instead of
kapok.

When you do not understand a symptom, look for an
allergy.

Bronchitis is an infection, usually bacterial, of the bronchial tubes. The cough and wheeze that accompany it may
sound like an asthma attack, but the other characteristics—
some fever (usually at least 100°), green or yellow mucus, and
a response to antibiotics—give away the infectious nature of
the problem.

Certainly asthmatics can get a secondary infection, since
allergy predisposes to infection, and many infections will trigger an allergy. If the infection seems to be a constant problem (if antibiotics are always necessary to get the patient
well), one should consider the use of vaccines of dead bacteria
(the patient's own or a stock solution) to desensitize the patient who is allergic to his own bacteria.

A fairly typical story is that of the baby who has been
well for six to ten months but becomes sick with a cold, cough,

and then bronchitis after the mother stops nursing him and he has just cut a tooth (two stresses). He is now into Level III; if nothing is done he will get sicker.

Stop the milk, up his vitamin C (to 200 to 500 mg per day) and his vitamin A (to 10,000 to 20,000 units per day), and give him a month or two. If he is well, you have moved him out of the dangerous level; keep up the minimum amounts to prevent recurrence. If he still keeps slipping into Level III and the doctor's office, the doctor should check his immune system (gamma globulin and white blood cell response) or the possibility of cystic fibrosis, a foreign body in the lungs, or a congenital lung anomaly (tracheoesophageal fistula, bronchostenosis, and so on). Allergy tests might be next.

If he seems to be doing well enough on the maintenance dose and gets a fresh cold and slight cough, don't wait to see if he is still in Level III. Begin immediately with 200 to 1000 mg, depending on age and fever, of vitamin C every hour or two. In twenty-four hours the condition should be improved enough for you to know that you will hold him at that level. Continue for another day at those high levels to clinch it, then reduce the vitamin C doses over the next five to seven days to the old sustaining dose.

Colds are virus infections characterized by a water discharge; they last about seven days. In children the first three days may be accompanied by fever but it is usually easily, although temporarily, controlled by aspirin (one grain per ten pounds of body weight every three or four hours) and comfortable hot baths. Colds, however, allow secondary bacterial infections to become superimposed. A Level I child becomes a Level II child if he gets a cold and slips into Level III, or even IV if he gets sick enough to require the doctor to treat him. A stress can get all this started, especially if there is fever and loss of appetite. At the first sign of a sneeze or a watery nose, the vitamin C dose should be increased (as noted in Bronchitis, p. 77). There is controversy about the beneficial effects of using vitamin C in colds and respiratory infections, as advocated by Dr. Linus Pauling and others. In one study, reported in the *Journal* of the American Medical Association in 1975, the investigating doctor found no difference in a large double-blind study using vitamin C for colds; however, he used no patients who had allergies. This would tend to corroborate the efficiency of the use of vitamin C, but it doesn't work on everybody. C seems to work better in those with allergies. It *does* have an antihistaminic effect. If you find it helps, you probably have an allergy. The antiviral effect of vitamin C apparently is related to its ability to enhance the formation of interferon, a natural antiviral substance.

If C doesn't work, you may not be taking enough, or your adrenals are really in trouble, or some mineral is not being provided in the diet, or the vitamin A intake is inadequate, or you are eating junk, or milk or food is the villain, or all of the above. But just because a lot of kids get colds, it does not follow that colds are a normal part of life. Don't give up!

It may be helpful to know that if one takes extra vitamin C for a cold and bronchitis follows, it may mean that he is more likely to benefit from vitamin A.

Vitamin B$_6$ (50 to 200 mg per day) may help the immune system get going; calcium (1000 to 2000 mg per day) plus vitamin D (1000 units per day) for a few days may help slow the cold symptoms. Vitamin E (100 to 800 units per day) helps vitamin A do its job.

For babies some have found the following helpful: one teaspoon of vitamin C powder in 3 ounces (about 100 cc) water, plus some lemon juice and a little honey to take the bite out. One teaspoon of this will provide about 100 mg of vitamin C and can be given every one to two hours for a day or two.

But a cold is a cold. You may be stuck with it, but if it lasts longer than a week and the mucus stays clear, it is surely an allergic rhinitis. If the discharge turns green or yellow, it is surely a secondary bacterial infection, and the owner of the cold is at least at health Level III.

Hay fever is the name for allergic rhinitis, the itchy, watery nose that is heralded by sneezing. The chronicity and the clarity of the discharge plus the sneeze make it an inhalation allergy. If postnasal drip and a zonking sound are prominent and there is little or no sneezing, the clear discharge usually makes one suspect a food allergy—most likely milk, but also possibly wheat, eggs, corn, potatoes, or citrus fruits.

Children often signal the world that they have a nasal allergy by rubbing, picking, sniffing, or putting fingers or foreign objects up their nostrils. Allergic shiners (black or purple discoloration of the lower eyelids), facial pallor, and hyponasality form a symptom group now called tension-fatigue syndrome, which almost always is due to drinking pasteurized-homogenized milk. (It is not always clear whether the culprit is the milk or what has been done to the milk, since many people can drink raw certified milk and not suffer thus.) It takes about three weeks of a diet free of milk for these clues to disappear, while the person with an inhalation allergy to house dust may clear up in two to five days of dust control.

If our Level I baby is being nursed satisfactorily and begins to sneeze, note what objects or animals are in the room at that moment and also think of what foods, milk, or drugs were ingested by the mother in the previous six to twelve hours . Then increase the vitamin C intake to 100 mg three or four times a day for a baby one to six months old. It might control an allergy, but you also don't know if it is a cold. Sometimes you can nip it in the bud. The relationship of an allergic phenomenon to the foods the nursing mother is ingesting has important predictive benefits. Many mothers will quit nursing on the assumption that the problem is their breast milk per se, when actually the problem is the allergen that is transported by the breast milk. Then, when it is discovered after a few days on cow's milk that the baby has a full-blown cow's-milk allergy, it is usually too late to get back to the breast. Some mothers experiment first by giving the baby cow's milk straight from the bottle, and if phlegm, snort, sneeze, wheeze, and rhinitis are fairly obviously related, she knows that nursing is the best, the safest, and she will go on with it for many months so her baby won't slip down a level. She also knows she had better get her 2 grams (2000 mg) of calcium from bone meal or dolomite and not from the cow. Also she discontinues taking or giving any colored, flavored vitamins.

But if the hay fever goes on despite milk changes and control of environmental dust and danders, one would suspect the Level II baby is becoming a Level III baby. Antihistamines and decongestants are worthwhile to see if temporary relief can be obtained. If they work, one can assume that an allergy is in progress, and that the child's adrenal glands are struggling. Vitamin C, B complex (especially B_6 and pantothenic acid), and vitamins A and E are all worthwhile. (See Allergy Program, above.)

A great many secondary infections (sinusitis, otitis, bronchitis, laryngitis, and tonsillitis) seem to have their antecedents in this seemingly benign watery nose, and a little effort extended in the first year or two may save the family much surgical and financial stress in the years to come. The chronic drip and phlegm not only make these tissues susceptible to infection but also seem to play a role in the enlargement of tonsils and adenoids. These latter lymphoid tissues seem to act like sponges, soaking up the mucus to the extent that they become obstructive. The deafness, mouth breathing, and crowded teeth that may result can cause the child to have his tonsils and adenoids removed and then require braces. All because he had an allergy to milk or house dust as an infant!

Statistics of patients with allergic rhinitis indicate that 25 percent of the children get worse (asthma), 50 percent stay the same, and 25 percent recover. The early warning sign of the watery nose and sneeze should encourage parents to try a few safe remedies.

Hoarseness suggests a problem in the larynx. Some babies are born with floppy vocal cords and their breathing is like a sail catching a breeze; it sounds scary, but if the child is pink and can sleep he will outgrow it in time.

The gradual increase of raspy breathing in a baby would suggest an allergic postnasal drip. If there is much sneezing, an inhalation allergy is suggested. If little or no sneezing is present, then a cow's-milk allergy should be considered (*see* Hay fever, above). Allergy control, milk changes, and the Stress Formula make sense. The baby has slipped a level or two and could be susceptible to more severe respiratory problems.

A sudden onset of hoarseness, especially accompanied by a barky cough, signals the croup. This is usually a virus inflammation of the larynx with little or no fever and occurs in the middle of a cold, dry winter night. Holding the child upright, plus giving him lemon juice and honey (with or without gin) as a cough remedy, should allow him to sleep for an hour or two between the twenty-minute barking sessions. If the child cannot sleep, if there is a fever above 102°, and especially if the child is bluish, oxygen and possibly a tracheal tube in the hospital are called for. This latter condition is bacterial epiglottitis and has lethal possibilities. Croup is a virus infection. The two conditions are two levels apart; one does not necessarily lead to the other.

Frequent croupy, barky attacks requiring steam and cough remedies usually suggest an underlying allergy. Bacterial epiglottitis usually means a poorly functioning immune system that cannot handle the stress of a cold, dry winter day and allows a germ to invade.

Croup that recurs is a Level III problem. It should be countered with the allergy environmental controls, no milk, and the Stress Formula. Epiglottitis does not allow enough time for nutritional treatment; it is a Level V medical emergency. *Don't stay at home poking vitamin C down a blue child; get him hospitalized.* Certainly the stress of the illness increases his need for vitamin C and B_6 and calcium, so these should be given intravenously or intramuscularly in the hospital along with oxygen and steam, an antibiotic, and maybe a tracheotomy. All the doctor has to do is write an order for 1000 mg of vitamin C and 100 mg of B_6 (intravenously) on the line following "oxygen and steam" and "check blood pressure, pulse, and respiration every 15 minutes." These children can die of adrenal gland exhaustion just as fast as if they had meningitis. It takes eight to twelve hours for the antibiotics to kill enough germs to relieve the symptoms and reduce the epiglottal swelling. The oxygen, steam, rest, tubation, and vitamins are just a holding action while the antibiotic is working. Some therapists have found that cortisone is effective in countering the tremendous inflammation of the epiglottis; it certainly should be considered if the child is deteriorating thirty to sixty minutes after the initial therapy has begun.

Once the child has recovered he may seem none the worse for wear, but his adrenals certainly will be tired. A Level IV Stress Formula should be instituted to build him back to a more relaxed II or III level. One attack does not make him immune; he could be *more* susceptible to this or some other nasty infection when a new stress hits him.

Influenza is the name attached to the viral respiratory infection that appears rather suddenly with fever, headache, scratchy windpipe, watery rhinitis, and generalized aching.

Some immune system has slipped and the "virus that is going around" invades. Three full days of fever and several days of choke and strangle are the rule—ten days total. If the discharge turns green or yellow, if the fever does not respond to aspirin (one grain per ten pounds of body weight every three to four hours) and hot baths and lasts for more than seventy-two hours, and if the cough gets tighter rather than looser after the third day, or if the disease is still present after twelve to fourteen days, it almost always means that a bacterial infection has superimposed itself and that some investigative or anti-biotic therapy is probably worthwhile. There has been a shift from Level III to Level IV.

When the phlegm settles, the flu victim must re-evaluate his or her lifestyle, job stress factors, nutrition, vitamin supplements, sleep, and recreation. Something allowed the body to become susceptible. Try to get back to Level II by the use of the Prevention Diet, plus the Stress Formula, plus the anti-infection routine.

Lymph nodes, those in the upper part of the neck tucked under the corner of the jawbone, usually swell if the throat or tonsils are infected. They are hard to find in a small baby because his neck is so short and fat, but it is worthwhile palpating them now and then, since they are an early warning sign of throat problems, especially tonsil infections.

Lymph tissues in children, including the tonsils, adenoids, and other lymph glands, usually swell somewhat for about six years and then shrink. This is the normal pattern and is probably related to the development of the person's immune system. Large glands that appear early or persistently after this initial swelling are considered a sign of a chronic infection; in the case of these anterior cervical nodes (just below the angle of the jaw bone), they indicate a chronic tonsillar infection. The tonsils are assumed to have bacteria (or viruses) entrapped in them, and the protein material that is stimulated thereby migrates to these local glands, which filter the material and are stimulated in turn to produce lymphocytes. The object of this mechanism, apparently, is to protect the body from invasion by this material (*see* Tonsillitis, p. 91).

If the bearer is sick, especially with a fever, and has an elevated white blood count, an antibiotic for ten days would be in order. It also gives a clue that this is suddenly a Level III or IV child and that the anti-infection program appropriate for age and level should be started simultaneously with the antibiotic. If nothing is done and the infection is a strep, it is possible that rheumatic fever (rare under age seven) or glomerulonephritis (more commonly seen in two- to five-year-olds) could ensue.

Mononucleosis is a virus infection which primarily involves the lymph tissues (tonsils, glands, and spleen). It can also cause liver swelling and a severe headache and consequently be confused with encephalitis or meningitis. Because young people are most likely to get mono, it is called the kissing disease, though unkissed youths can get it too.

A more logical explanation of its occurrence in young people is that they are growing fast, often eating poorly, and frequently living under stress, thus this ubiquitous virus finds easy access to unprotected cells. A healthy body should not become a host to this disease.

If someone falls prey to mononucleosis, he or she should be given 1000 mg of vitamin C every one to two hours along with the Stress Formula. If there is doubt whether it is mono or a streptococcal throat infection, a throat culture might be taken. Penicillin or erythromycin would be given if it is a strep, but in either case the big doses of vitamin C would be helpful.

Mono lasts a month, but this can be shortened to two weeks if the anti-infection and Stress Formulas are used. This is desirable, since prolonged bed rest allows leg-muscle wastage and bone decalcification. I am impressed by how short the disease and the convalescence become when an injection of vitamin C and the B complex is given soon after the diagnosis is made. (Vitamin C, 4 grams; calcium gluconate, one gram; and B_6, 100 mg intravenously may be dramatic.)

Mouth breathing is usually caused by a nasal obstruction due to an allergy which makes the nasal tissues swell up. Frequent offenders are pollens and danders from grass, trees, wool, feathers, and animals (*see* Hay fever, Chapter 5). Milk can cause this hyponasality (*see* Tension-fatigue syndrome, below). Large adenoids can become obstructive (*see* Tonsillitis, Chapter 5). Foreign bodies up the nose can cause this (*see* Bad breath, Chapter 5). A broken nose might make it difficult to breathe out of one side. A virus cold will do it.

A look up the nose at the mucous membranes may be helpful in deciding what course of action to take. Pale, slightly bluish, swollen tissues will suggest an inhalant as the cause. A fairly normal appearance would suggest the obstruction is farther back (swelling due to milk allergy or large adenoids). A greenish-yellow, slightly bloody, putrid-smelling discharge from one side is supposed to be the sign of a foreign body up the nose. A previously broken nose frequently is revealed by a deviated septum.

A nose plugged from a cold or flu is pink and red inside and the secretions are clear. A purulent rhinitis causes redness and crusts up the nose, and the discharge is green or yellow.

We have nutrition programs for all these conditions, but the doctor may be needed if it is a foreign body up the nose or a deviated septum. If the allergy-control program does not help and noisy breathing continues, especially at night, then the adenoids may have to come out.

Orthodontists believe that hyponasality and allergies and mouth breathing all contribute to a poorly developed lower jaw. The child simply lets his mouth hang open. He hates to chew because he finds it hard to breathe while eating. He consumes large amounts of liquid calories and soft foods, and so becomes an even likelier candidate for dental attention. So be forewarned: a chronic mouth-breathing child runs the risk of future orthodontia. Telling him to shut his mouth is not enough.

Pneumonia can be viral or bacterial. Usually a spiking chill and fever come rapidly with or without a cold or slight cough. A Level I or II person may plunge to Level V in one hour. He must get to the doctor or the hospital. An x-ray, culture, and blood count should tell if bacteria or viruses are causative, and appropriate antibiotics can be ordered. Along with supportive hospital techniques, it is worthwhile to use vitamin C (1000 mg every one to three hours intravenously) and the B complex (50 mg of each plus 100 mg of B_6). There are two reasons for this approach: first, the absence of these nutrients may have allowed the sickness to begin with; second, the disease now puts further stress on the liver and lungs and adrenals, and these vitamins would provide the body with the wherewithal to help fight the infection.

As with other severe infections, the victim must reorganize his lifestyle, his diet, and his nutrients to get himself out of that dangerous level. A trip to the Caribbean may not be enough.

Rhinitis is a runny nose. Allergic rhinitis is the watery drip accompanied by sneezing and itchiness (*see* Hay fever, p. 80). Someone might have been in Level I, but these symptoms would put him into Level II right away. He must get rid of the cat or pillow, get out of the ragweed, and use the antiallergic program, otherwise he might slip into Level III because of the development of asthma, bronchitis, sinusitis, otitis, or a secondary bacterial infection. It's also possible that the rhinitis could become permanent.

If the secretions turn green or yellow, a bacterial infection has occurred, and more heroic nutrition or antibiotics are called for. Fever and headache would suggest a visit to the doctor.

Skin testing for pollen, house dust, grass, and trees is worthwhile to determine what to eliminate or what should be put into a vaccine for the weekly shots to desensitize the patient. Frequently the victim's room can be made dust-free and an antihistamine given for temporary relief while the sufferer is building up the assumed-to-be-exhausted adrenal glands. It may take six to eighteen months to slow down the symptoms by using the basic adrenal support Stress Formula program plus the antiallergic nutrients, but the relief may be more complete (and even cheaper) than the allergy-desensitizing shots—which may take the same length of time. Many people take advantage of both the medical and the nutritional approaches, one being supportive of the other. Try to avoid cortisone.

A constant purulent discharge may be further helped by cutting out all dairy products plus periodic injections of a dead bacterial vaccine (the patient's or a stock solution).

Sinusitis is a bacterial infection of a sinus. Infants have poorly developed sinuses, so this condition is usually not a problem until age three to six. It has to be initiated by an allergy which allows for swollen tissue to plug up the opening to the sinus; also, there has to be a secondary infection (green

or yellow discharge) to qualify. It probably needs an antibiotic (usually ampicillin for a child less than five years old
and penicillin over that age), especially if a fever is present.
But if recognized in time it may respond in a day or two to
vitamin C (500 mg every two hours for two days for those
under five years and 1000 mg every two hours for the older
child or adult). If this doesn't work or if bronchitis appears,
one should have used big doses of vitamin A (100,000 to
200,000 units per day for three or four days) or an antibiotic.
One has now slipped into Level III, and upon recovery (and
to prevent a recurrence) the Stress Formula as well as an
allergy investigation must be initiated or the problem will
recur.

Sneezing is a clue that the sneezer has inhaled an irritant; for some this is possible in the bright sun or on taking a
glass of milk. Some allergy-prone people recognize sneezing
as the harbinger of an allergy attack, a cold, stress, or a visit
from a creditor or an in-law. Instead of waiting to see what
is coming, a prudent person should realize that a new and
potentially dangerous level has been reached and the stress
or allergy program should be initiated.

Vitamin C, B_6, and pantothenic acid should be taken
relentlessly for two to three days in an effort to abort whatever
it is. Antihistamines and decongestants are compatible with
the above and could provide comfort. "Feeding a cold" may
be justified; the body is on the verge of a sickness and needs
to be nourished. Waiting to see if one gets a sinusitis, a bronchitis, or an asthma attack does not seem like a bright idea.

A sneeze is like a Geiger counter; the more one sneezes,
the more likely the irritant is nearby. It also has to mean that
the victim is susceptible to allergies. If only one person in the
family drips and sneezes near the cat, it is possible with nutri-

tion to build up a tolerance to cat fur and dander. If everyone in the house sneezes when the cat is nearby, the cat should be given away.

Tension-fatigue syndrome is a combination of symptoms and signs that leads to a diagnosis of allergy, usually to a food, and usually to homogenized, pasteurized cow's milk with its additives. The children (or adults) with this syndrome usually are fair people with blue or green eyes, so the dark-blue lower eyelids are in sharp contrast to the pale cheeks. Some parents believe that since the whole family looks like that, it is hereditary. Not so. The allergy is hereditary, but not the washed-out look. Most of these people have postnasal drip and make an almost continuous sniffing–snorting–throat-clearing sound (zonking). It is as if they feel a bunch of rubber bands hanging down their throat and are trying to clear it. They frequently complain of stomachaches and headaches and generalized fatigue. Various muscle aches and pains complete the picture.

It usually takes about two to three weeks of avoidance of all dairy products, or whatever particular food they are allergic to, to clear up the syndrome. Allergy testing is not reliable to discover the offender. A story of milk allergy (skin, respiratory, or intestinal) in the past, plus ear and tonsillar infections is usually enough to suggest that milk is the likely cause.

Some people find that raw milk or goat's milk will not cause this syndrome, which suggests that the processing of milk or the additives are at fault. Some doctors find that the allergy-control program allows the milk to be consumed without producing the phlegm.

Tonsillectomy and *adenoidectomy* are being done less often now as a result of a number of studies. (In one study children aged four to five years were put on the waiting list for the T & A operation. In six to twelve months when the time to operate had arrived it was discovered that at least half of them no longer required the surgery.) The operation carries an inherent risk, as all operations do. If the child can be "held together" with good nutrition and possibly antibiotics, the tonsil and adenoid tissues tend to shrink after age six and become less obstructive. Some children develop asthma after a tonsillectomy, as if the tonsils were protecting the lungs (or if the stress of the surgery allowed an allergy to develop). But some children, on the other hand, are relieved of asthma after the removal of the tonsils.

Tonsils and adenoids should not get large enough to become obstructive. Frequent sore throats and ear infections indicate an allergic condition (usually to milk). If a child under one or two years of age can be made resistant to infections and allergies with a no-milk, no-sugar routine and the Stress Formula, the tonsils and adenoids may not swell to the point of becoming obstructive or chronically infected.

The most common indication for tonsillectomy is obstructive breathing during sleep when the rather pendulous tonsils flop down in the throat. Such tonsils should be removed. Adenoids are removed if they are gross enough to plug up the Eustachian tubes and the child is continualy deaf because of chronic otitis media. If his hearing is impaired, his sound perception is jeopardized to the point that speech and communication in general are defective.

Awareness of the problem and early nutritional intervention may preclude a stressful operation. (*See* Tension-fatigue syndrome, above, *and* Otitis media, Chapter 6.)

Tonsillitis is the inflammation of the tonsils. A virus is most likely to be the cause of this fairly common problem, but a streptococcus may invade and if not properly treated may lead to one or a number of nasty complications, including glomerulonephritis, rheumatic fever, an abscess behind the tonsil, septicemia, and pneumonia. It is now considered mandatory to culture red tonsils when they are accompanied by fever and swollen neck glands to determine the presence of the strep. If strep is found, full doses of penicillin (or erythromycin) are used for ten days. If not, just the standard "fluid, aspirin, and rest" are recommended.

One doctor stated that he had never seen a strep sore throat in non-milk drinkers. Many of us would doubt that, but it does suggest that allergies can produce a susceptibility to bacterial invasion. In either case, virus or bacterial, effort should be made to move a Level III throat patient to a safer level: by controlling allergies, by upping the daily vitamin C and B complex to double the preinfection level for a couple of months, and maybe by increasing the vitamin A to 50,000 units for a few weeks.

During the course of the infection, whether it is treated with an antibiotic or not, the anti-infection routine should be followed: lots of juices, no sugary drinks, and as much nutritious food as possible should be urged down the reluctant throat. Rest is okay until the fever is under 100° for a day, and then activity must be encouraged. Lying in bed prolongs convalescence and allows the leg muscles to atrophy and the bones to decalcify. Bed rest does not prevent complications; it may even encourage them. □

If your child is to have surgery, bring some protein snack to the operating room—not for you, but for the surgeon.

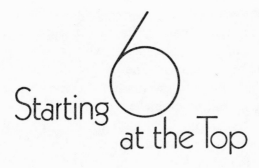

Starting at the Top

The skull houses some of the most delicate and precious mechanisms of the human body, including the brain and the sense organs of sight, hearing, and smell. In my patients I see much needless impairment of these crucial systems—teeth rotted due to poor hygiene and ingestion of sweets, hearing lost due to repeated ear infections, sight weakened by prenatal malnutrition.

While the newborn's endowments in these areas are largely inherited, much can be done to keep the perfect ones healthy and the less perfect ones at the best possible level of efficiency. Above all, don't be careless about maintaining these systems in good order. Once the damage is done, it's done permanently.

Ears and Eyes

Blindness may be caused by injury, infection (congenital rubella, retrolental fibroplasia, syphilis, toxoplasmosis), malnutrition (vitamin A deficiency usually), galactosemia, brain injury, and disuse (following uncorrected crossed eyes).

Some of these are avoided by good nutrition and preventive care. For example, retrolental fibroplasia is almost exclusively seen in premature babies who required extra oxygen to prevent brain injury. The oxygen seems to stimulate blood vessels in the eye to proliferate; the vessels then thrombose and scar, occluding retinal reception. Had the mother practiced good nutrition during pregnancy, she might have had a nine-month baby. In addition, "preemies" are known to be low in vitamin E, which suggests that E might prevent this problem.

Crossed eyes might be related to faulty prenatal nutrition. The infant cannot establish binocular vision, because his cortex perceives a double image. His brain then suppresses the image it gets from one eye; this is called suppression blindness, or amblyopia ex anopsia.

Blind people frequently rock back and forth. This action could be the response of the brain to inadequate messages from the sense organs (eyes) as to where the body is in space. The stimulation of the semicircular canals in the inner ear may help the brain decide (without the use of eyes) if the body is upright. Some blind people do not need to rock when they take large doses of the B vitamins (orally or by injection). This calming effect suggests that the brain may be under some kind of stress either from the blindness or from the condition that caused the blindness.

Vitamin A-deficient blindness is rare in the United States, which may be the result of good nutrition or the inability of the medical profession to recognize a subclinical form. But surveys indicate that the North American diet is deficient in carotene and vitamin A, so night blindness, at least, would be the problem with some of the people who stumble about at twilight. Those who do not take vitamin supplements, who work under bright lights, who notice "tired" eyes after reading, who have rough skin on thighs and upper arms and possibly respiratory infections, might be suffering from a lack of vitamin A sufficient to allow the above symptoms but not severe enough to cause actual structural eyeball changes.

If any or all of the above indications are present, a month of a vitamin A intake of 100,000 units per day would be enough to improve everything without running the risk of toxicity. Obviously, attention to the diet would be appropriate; carrots (tops and bottom), and liver should be in the diet frequently.

Deafness or *hearing loss* in a child is usually due to the fluid left behind the eardrum after a bout of otitis media. Sometimes the drum is retracted because the Eustachian tube (the passageway between the upper pharynx and the middle ear which allows for equalization of air pressure on both sides of the drum) is obstructed (allergies, adenoids) and the air in the middle ear space is absorbed, leaving a vacuum. A tube may have to be placed in the drum to allow it to resume its normal position; air is necessary on both sides of the drum to allow it to vibrate when sound waves strike it. Sometimes a thick gluelike secretion must be sucked out of the middle ear to allow the drum to vibrate freely. Many children have had a hearing loss since birth and have no way of comparing their hearing ability with the normal. Auditory screening tests in early childhood are a valuable preschool procedure, especially if there is a history of ear infection or poor speech development in the first year (*see* Otitis media, below).

Many children are deaf as a result of the mother contracting rubella in the first trimester of the pregnancy. The virus apparently invades and destroys the acoustical nerves carrying the impulses to the brain. Destroyed nerves cannot be revived, but it is possible that some of the nerves are only damaged and could be partially functional if supplied the proper nutrients. Preventing rubella by the use of the rubella vaccine in girls well before the child-bearing years should be a part of the shot schedule in childhood. It would do no harm, and might be beneficial, to give large amounts of the Stress Formula to any pregnant woman exposed to rubella. If she contracts it in the first few months and elects not to have a therapeutic abortion, she should at least increase her intake of the Stress Formula in the hope that her unborn may be less involved. There has to be a reason why some babies have severe damage to ears, eyes, and brain and others are not affected at all. Nutrition might be the key to this difference.

Parents report that their deaf children are more "active" than the nonaffected siblings. The stress of the illness might produce this sensitivity, or it might mean that the stress of an incomplete sensory awareness is responsible for the acuteness of tactile and visual stimuli.

Otitis media is a middle-ear infection. It is hard to understand why this should be so common in the modern child until one realizes that it is initiated by allergies—usually to cow's milk. The story goes almost always as follows: a mother has satisfactorily nursed her baby until seven or eight months of age. He cuts some teeth (a stress for both), she decides to quit nursing because it is painful and her doctor and her relatives encourage discontinuance. The baby develops a cold and in a few days runs a fever, the mucus runs green or yellow from his nose, and he cries in pain and bats at his ears. (A clue about ear infection: babies will continue to eat solids but won't suck if the eardrum is sore, because the vacuum thus created pulls on the eardrums, and this is very painful.)

One ear infection puts a child into the Level II health category and, of course, puts him at risk for another. If the cold-induced ear infection also can be related to some stress (teething, colds in the family, a move or injury) and one can prevent further stress, nothing need be done. If, however, there was a formula change within a reasonable period of time (two to six weeks), then one operates on the premise that the change allowed the allergy to appear. If a baby is under six to eight months of age, it is usually necessary to switch to soybean milk. If he is over this age and happens to like solids, try giving him water, juice, and extra calcium.

A Level III child for ear infection has already had three or four bouts of otitis media and the doctor is suggesting that tubes be placed in his eardrums to equalize the pressure—and possibly that his tonsils and adenoids should be removed.

Once the tonsils and adenoids swell sufficiently to cause bouts of otitis media, hyponasal breathing, and swollen glands in the neck, it is usually too late to reverse the process by eliminating milk or other allergens. It may be prudent to remove these obstructive tissues, but a three-month trial program of the Prevention Diet, no dairy products, control of house and pet allergies, plus the Stress and anti-infection formulas might save the child from another stress.

In Level IV a child would be partially deaf as a result of repeated ear infections that caused retraction of the eardrum or residual fluid behind his ear drums. A visit to the ear-nose-and-throat doctor is a must for relief of these problems, which is usually achieved by surgery. The difficult thing to accept is that in spite of all this operative intervention, the child can still get ear infections. When this happens, the ENT doctor usually sends the patient to an allergist; one wonders why allergy was not even thought of earlier.

A Level V child for ear trouble has a permanent perforation in his eardrum, has permanent hearing loss due to the scarring of the tissues in the middle ear, or has infected mastoids. Even in these days of antibiotics, these complications are not unusual. Why? we must ask, when it probably could have been prevented by taking action at the first sign.

Mouth and Teeth

Aphthous stomatitis is a virus mouth infection usually heralded by a fever in a one- to two-year-old child who has been previously well. The fever and headache last about three days, at which time the child feels better but then starts to drool and refuses to eat. A good look in the mouth reveals several blossoming canker sores, which take the standard five to seven days to heal. Hunger usually forces the child to eat some soft, nonacid food or drink, but some stubborn kids will just sit there for the week crying and drooling and flirting with dehydration. It is important to note urinary output; a minimum of two wet diapers a day should mean the child will be spared a hospital visit and intravenous fluids.

Because there is no antibiotic for a virus infection, the parents should not wait for the third day to discover the nature of the disease; they should start the regime for fever at the first sign of the illness (*see* Anti-Infection Program, Chapter 3) or at least get the child started on the fluids. They should aim for a two- to three-quart fluid intake plus a two- to five-gram intake of vitamin C. The vitamin C might shorten the disease to three or four days.

Bleeding gums are supposed to be an indication of scurvy, but gum infection from bacteria or virus is another possible cause. Injury or tooth eruption may also cause an oozing of blood. Because vitamin C helps fight infection and encourages healing, the daily dose should be doubled for any of the above indications. If simple tooth-brushing causes bleeding and if increasing the vitamin C does not control the "pink toothbrush" sign, some dental or medical evaluation should be made of the rest of the body to discover the cause.

Canker sores are considered a virus infection following a local injury or some stress situation, such as the onset of a menstrual period, the ingestion of walnuts, chocolate, or citrus, or the experience of some emotional stress. At the very first sign of the pesky sore just inside the edge of the lip or on the inside of the cheek or where the cheek joins the gum, one might stop its progress by the ingestion of pantothenic acid, 100 mg for a child and 500 mg for an adult. This dose every hour or two for the next six to twelve hours may control it completely or at least shorten the otherwise miserable seven-day course.

If recurrences of canker sores continue, one must look to and change his stressful lifestyle, his diet, or perhaps increase his daily dose of pantothenic acid. Canker sores are an early warning sign that all is not well. If pantothenic acid helps, it suggests that the adrenal glands are not being nourished properly or are being stressed beyond their capacity to recuperate. Some find 1000 mg of vitamin C four times a day will arrest the sores. Alfalfa tablets, sprouts and legumes are good sources of pantothenic acid.

Caries, or *tooth decay,* is a clue that the bearer has been poorly nourished during some past period of his life. In some babies, the teeth erupt misshapen, pitted, and stained and seem to rot almost immediately. This is a clue that the mother was malnourished for a number of vitamins and minerals during the pregnancy. Weston Price notes in his book *Nutrition and Physical Degeneration* that primitive people, no matter what their geographical location, had only two to four cavities per one hundred teeth (average one cavity in every third person), had nicely rounded dental arches (no crowded teeth and little malocclusion), and never needed removal of wisdom teeth. As soon as sugar and refined flour came to these people through increased trade and better transportation, the cavity rate increased and crowded teeth, high-arched palate, and long narrow faces began to appear.

Plaque formation, because it is the precursor of cavities, requires preventive flossing and more efficient brushing and coarse foods to chew. Instead of drinking apple juice, we should eat the apple plus the core. Cavities follow a poor diet; we should imitate our stone age forefathers.

The mother's diet before the baby is born, then, may be as important as the diet of the child throughout life. Dr. Price noted an increased incidence of skeletal problems after the refined foods were ingested: flat feet and leg, knee, hip, and pelvic abnormalities. Because of narrow pelvises in girls born of poorly nourished mothers, there appeared to be an increased need for Caesarean sections.

A Level I child obviously would be so well nourished (because his mother ate well and had no stress during her pregnancy) that his baby teeth at least would be white, clean, and free of cavities. He might slip to a Level II for caries if a tooth decayed. It should be filled, but some attention must be paid to the diet—stop the junk and up the minerals (calcium, magnesium, and maybe phosphorus) and B vitamins.

A new cavity every few months means that not enough is being done.

If he still slips into Level III or IV (two or three cavities a year), he is in real trouble and perhaps should be evaluated more thoroughly for some other hidden problem. A hair analysis might reveal some odd deficiencies in minerals, which should be provided to correct the problem.

A gum boil which results from an apical abscess puts one into Level V for caries. This really gets serious, since the infection could spread to the heart or kidneys. Whopping doses of vitamin C (5 to 20 grams a day), plus appropriate antibiotics, might slow the devastation.

It seems quite logical to cut out the sugar and white flour from our diets just from the standpoint of the known relationship to dental caries. Why do parents allow sugar in the house when they know that cavities will surely follow?

Fluoride and tooth brushing and flossing are not enough; they are holding actions, and not very good ones at that. The simplest, cheapest, and most effective cure is to get rid of the sugar.

We do have taste buds for sweetness, but the only things humans need to taste that are sweet are breast milk and fruit (the latter only to assure that we will get some vitamin C). Even breast milk can rot out the teeth if the baby is allowed to nurse all night—using the breast as a pacifier. Fruit and honey are cavity-inducing and should be consumed along with nuts or raw vegetables, which tend to cleanse the enamel.

Fluoridation of the water supply may not be the universal simple answer to tooth decay. There is no doubt that it helps form a tough, decay-resistant enamel on the teeth, but the basis of its use has been somewhat misinterpreted. Deaf Smith County, in the Panhandle of West Texas, for instance, has a soil full of calcium and magnesium carbonate and about two parts per million of fluoride. This particular combination produces water and plants that when consumed have an anti-cavity effect.

To believe that just putting fluoride in the water supply will protect the teeth is possibly naïve and may be dangerous, at least to some. There are many sensitive people who get sick when they drink fluoridated water. This may be because the fluoride acts as an enzyme depressant when not combined with calcium and magnesium. Taking dolomite and eating no sugar or white flour seems a safer way to handle the caries problem, whether your water supply is fluoridated or not. Fluoridate sugar, not water.

Cheilosis is the name given to the cracks that appear at the corners of the mouth. Dry weather, stress, food allergy, borderline vitamin B intake might all contribute. If the sores become infected and spread with the formation of yellow crusts, impetigo is now superimposed and some antibiotic ointment would be appropriate. Because of the danger of sensitization, it is best to use an antibiotic that will not also be used internally.

Stop milk, chocolate, citrus fruit, tomatoes, and any relatively new food. Follow the Stress Formula. A clue: rashes or pimples about the mouth or face are usually due to a food if there are corresponding spots about the anal opening or scattered over the buttocks.

If sores still resist healing, chelated zinc, 50 to 100 mg per day, should be added to the diet.

Pyorrhea is the end stage of poor mouth hygiene. Swollen, tender, infected gums that bleed when barely touched or brushed soon lead to loose teeth. This is an emergency situation and requires 5 to 10 grams of vitamin C daily plus stress amounts of B complex vitamins and the Prevention Diet. Bone meal or dolomite to provide 2000 mg of calcium would help, and vitamin A (50,000 units per day) should slow down the deterioration, if it can be helped, in about two to three weeks.

Taste distortion is called *dysgeusia* and is usually due to a zinc deficiency. When it is severe, the victim believes the food he is trying to choke down tastes like feces. Eating becomes a problem. Within two weeks of starting 100 mg zinc supplement (chelated is best), the taste perceptions become normal again.

It is possible that the reluctant-to-eat two- to four-year-old might be suffering from a zinc deficiency. Many white spots in the nails would tend to support the diagnosis. The incidence of zinc deficiency seems to be rising, because much of the zinc has been washed out of the topsoil in the United States and is not being replaced. Kelp from the ocean seems to be a natural way to replace this loss. Kelp powder as a seasoning should be a daily addition to the diet.

Teeth grinding is usually considered a sign of tension or anxiety, but it can come from any distress. The child, in an effort to block out uncomfortable stimuli, grinds his teeth.

Pediatricians know that the most common cause of restless sleep and teeth grinding is pinworms (*see* Pinworms, Chapter 8). A child who seems susceptible to worm infestation is usually a thumb sucker or a nose-picker. Perhaps if he were optimally nourished he would not suck his thumb and not have an itchy, allergic nose, and as a consequence would be less likely to become infested by transferring the worm eggs to his mouth.

If the teeth grinding does not stop following prescription of a vermifuge, a trial of the no-milk, no-sugar Prevention Diet would be worthwhile. If this does not work, then calcium and magnesium (1000 mg calcium and 500 mg magnesium at bedtime) might have a calming effect. Extra B_6 (100 mg at bedtime) has been noted to have a quieting effect. Pantothenic acid, 300 to 500 mg a day has helped some.

A protein feeding at bedtime may prevent the fall of blood sugar during the night. In some people, the fall of blood sugar stimulates the adrenals to secrete adrenalin, and an uncomfortable sensation follows. As a compensation, the victim grinds his teeth. Stress obviously will produce the same adrenalin flow.

Thrush (*see* Candidiasis, Chapter 4) is a yeast infection in the mouth which looks like milk curds plastered to the tongue and cheeks. It is common in newborns delivered from mothers who have vaginal candidiasis.   □

The smartest thing a flight attendant can do with a hijacker is to feed him. Assume his neocortex has run out of energy and the lights are off in his conscience.

Body 7 Systems

The bones, muscles, and circulatory system form an infrastructure that is constantly in use. When these systems get in trouble they have painful ways of letting us know. Joints ache, muscles cramp, "tired" blood leaves us feeling punk. Yet—assuming things haven't gone too far—all these systems respond marvelously to the preventive approach of good nutrition and stress reduction. An added element should be a fairly active lifestyle. Avoid being sedentary. Get the kind of exercise that uses these systems in a healthy way. It will help keep the muscles in tone, the bones properly calcified, and the bloodstream unobstructed and elastic.

Walking, running, swimming, climbing should be a way of life that leads to chronic health. If the family eats nourishing food, it is easy to exercise because fatigue is no problem.

Bones are composed of calcium, phosphorus, magnesium, and a few trace elements and are held together with connective tissue that depends on vitamin C. Studies have indicated that all these elements are needed for healthy bones;

large amounts are obviously needed during the growing years, but if they are not continued throughout life the bones will demineralize, leading to backache and severe curvature in old age. Vitamin D picks up the calcium from the intestines and deposits it into the bones. A specific level of calcium floats around in the bloodstream for metabolic needs, to be available for blood-clotting, and it seems to have a specific calming effect on the nervous system. In general, the bones act as a reservoir of calcium; the vitamin D deposits it into the bones, as noted, and the parathyroid hormone works to remove the calcium from the bones and to put it into the bloodstream. The enzymes responsible for the production of the body's hormones need amino acids from well-balanced protein and the B complex vitamins.

Bone pain and muscle aches are signals that some element is in insufficient supply. A person thus afflicted would be served better by a sound diet and supplements of bone meal or dolomite and the B complex vitamins than he would by aspirin, which just treats the symptoms.

Muscles are chiefly protein, so amino acids are needed to build them. Potassium has to be supplied to permit contraction; a lack of potassium will cause profound weakness. (Many people notice weakness after taking diuretics, which promote potassium loss from the body through the kidneys. Potassium also is lost with diarrhea; this accounts for the weakness associated with intestinal flu.) A low-carbohydrate diet may lead to weakness because the muscles need glucose for fuel. Glycogen, the "starch" of the human body, is stored in the muscles for use between meals; the muscles will convert this to sugar when it is needed.

Muscle cramps after exercise usually are due to the accumulation of lactic acid. Calcium in sufficient amounts in the muscles and bloodstream will prevent these cramps. Tight, spastic muscles can be relieved by extra calcium.

Tetany (generalized muscle twitching) results from very low calcium levels—but this is the end stage of a severe deficiency, because the regulatory mechanism of the body normally will compensate for falling blood calcium by mobilizing calcium from the bones. A high phosphorus intake (animal protein) accompanied by decrease in milk intake could lead to a relative calcium deficiency, resulting in such problems as tight muscles, cramps, menstrual pain, nervousness, and hyperactivity. Most hyperactive children have low levels of calcium in their hair, despite adequate intakes of milk.

If milk and dairy-product intake must be curtailed because of allergic problems, dolomite (calcium and magnesium) or bone meal should be given daily (1000 mg calcium per day as powder or pills is just about right plus cod-liver oil at about the 500-to-1000 units level).

Stress depletes the body of calcium and bed rest allows the bones to demineralize; calcium and mineral intake should be increased after fractures and during pregnancy and nursing.

Anemia is thin, tired blood. In children it is usually the result of iron deficiency and is seen in those who consume cow's milk to the exclusion of iron-bearing solid foods (especially liver, meat, most fruits and vegetables). These children are pale, tired-acting, prone to sleep, and frequently sick. Pale cheeks, little color to the nailbeds or inner side of eyelids are clues, but a hemoglobin test confirms the low amount of circulating iron. This low level in the blood also means the iron stores in the body are low. Three months of supplemental iron is usually advisable.

A change of diet and an iron tonic is usually all that is necessary. Taking extra vitamin C (100 to 500 mg) with the iron (10 to 30 mg per day) makes it more readily absorbed. A few children have an intolerance to milk to the extent that dairy food ingestion causes microscopic hemorrhages along the intestinal tract; this slow blood loss will continue to keep the patient anemic until the milk is discontinued.

Other types of anemia affect the noniron parts of the red cell; copper, B_{12}, and folic-acid deficiencies may result. It would be best to get a specific diagnosis from a laboratory. Lead poisoning will lead to anemia, as will chronic infection. Vegetarians may not get enough B_{12}, and those on goat's milk may be low in folic acid.

A nutritional supplement or an adequate diet would prevent all this from happening to the blood in the first place.

Arthritis is rare in children, but is devastating when it occurs and may cause a lifetime disability.

Septic arthritis usually causes a high fever and exhaustion along with the severe pain and muscle contraction to guard the affected joint. The pus (usually the dreaded staphylococcus) in the joint space rapidly destroys the delicate lining tissues and must be aspirated. The affected joint is usually put at rest and traction applied to counteract the spasm of the muscles. Huge doses of antibiotics are given to kill these germs. Most patients do well, but cure is usually associated with some limitation of motion or chronic arthritis.

Infection is always a stress, so the patient must be supplied with huge amounts of vitamin C (5 to 10 grams per day) plus the B complex (200 mg of each of the Bs per day). If necessary, a parent should try to sit at the bedside of the child in the hospital and monitor the food being taken. In general, hospital food is usually loaded with "naked" carbohydrates.

Juvenile rheumatoid arthritis is considered an autoimmune disease (allergy to self) and suggests an insufficient excretion of the adrenal gland hormone, cortisol. The onset of the disease may be spiking fever, and it may be a year or two before the aching, swollen joints give a clue to the problem.

The doctor should be able to make the diagnosis with blood tests, and the Stress Formula should be started, but any fever would suggest the child has *some* disease process going on, and extra vitamin C would be mandatory.

Standard medical practice is physiotherapy and anti-inflammatory drugs (like aspirin) for the relief of pain. We now have other options, however (such as the Stress Formula), and one of our aims is to avoid using cortisone.

When arthritis occurs following a stress, it may well be the somatic manifestation of that stress, which may be emotional or nutritional or age-related.

A woman told me that during pregnancy with her second child, her first child died of leukemia. This stress so drained her that she was unable to nurse her new baby, who promptly developed a severe milk allergy with unremitting vomiting and diarrhea despite seven formula changes. He required weeks of hospitalization and intravenous feedings. At age four, this child now has severe, crippling rheumatoid arthritis.

The stress of her baby's death depleted this mother's adrenal glands and the adrenals of her unborn baby—who, having no protection from allergies, developed a severe allergy to milk. The stress of the condition would only serve to prolong and intensify the adrenal-gland exhaustion until some other organ system collapsed, in this case the joints.

The mother's obstetrician should have loaded her with the B and C vitamins—maybe double the Stress Formula. She should have been encouraged—or pushed—into nursing to forestall the cow's-milk allergy. When the milk allergy occurred, the baby should have been given injections of the B and C vitamins; this would have healed the eroded intestines as well as rebuilt the adrenals.

If the stiff joints and wasted muscles have already become established, it would not be too late to arrest the process and, if not too much damage has been done, to reverse it a little. Treatment would call for massive doses of vitamin C (5 to 10 grams for a child each day); all the B complex, up to 200 mg of each, plus pantothenic acid, 4 to 5 grams per day, and up to 500 mgl of B_6; perhaps 100,000 units of vitamin A per day for at least a month (headaches, irritability, scaly skin and hair loss would suggest a toxic dosage). Vitamin D would be important to get the calcium back into the bones; 1000 mg of calcium a day (dolomite or bone meal) should help to recalcify the bones and have a calming effect on the muscles and painful joints as well as allow more comfort so physiotherapy can be continued.

These patients don't want to move; it hurts too much. Disuse causes atrophy of muscles and decalcification of the bones; the calcium settles in the soft tissue of the joint or is washed out in the kidneys. (Kidney stones are common in sedentary people.) The patients must be exercised, despite their protests. No junk food at all is allowed. The slow growth and lack of exercise reduces the appetite, so every morsel has to be highly nutritious.

Everything possible must be done before someone puts these children on cortisone. The results of using vitamin C are under scrutiny. A recent study indicated antiarthritic benefits in this vitamin. Husky dogs were given vitamin C prophylactically and did not get the arthritis they seem prone to in spite of making their own vitamin C. Nevertheless, some people (and animals) have stress-related disease no matter how much vitamin C they get or have.

Backache (and muscle ache in general) is due to many things: overuse (lactic acid accumulation and calcium depletion); injury (blood leaking into muscles, resulting in pain); emotional stress (nerves cause a muscle spasm, muscle spasm causes pain fibers to send a message to the brain, which sends more messages back to muscles to go into more spasm—a vicious cycle); infections (polio, flu); and allergy (milk, corn, and the like).

It is truly amazing how something as cheap and safe as pantothenic acid (100 to 300 mg two to four times a day) will relieve almost all of the garden variety of muscle spasms due to strain and tension. It is thought that the pantothenic acid helps the adrenals to make cortisone, which promotes cell function and has a specific anti-inflammatory action, superior to aspirin.

Chiropractors are trained to "read" the body by feeling muscles. A spastic muscle suggests that a diseased organ or tissue has sent a message to the spinal-cord segment that innervates the muscle. Working the spasm out of the muscle may have a curative effect on the corresponding organ. If the spasm returns, the organ needs to be treated more directly.

I also wonder if the relief of the spasm doesn't have some calming effect on the neocortex, which is where psychosomatic problems start. Chiropractors are, in general, way ahead of medical doctors in the nutritional approach to treatment. They can feel a calcium deficit in the muscles (some firm muscle bands alternating with some softer ones) or a magnesium depletion (the muscle feels like corduroy under the skin). They may be closer to the patient and literally able to "feel" the difference between poorly nourished skin and muscle and optimally fed tissues.

Of course, if a week of pantothenic acid, a few chiropractic manipulations, and some extra calcium to relax the muscles (1000 mg per day) do nothing for the sore muscles, an x-ray seems prudent to check the state of the bones. If the bones check out all right, the condition suggests some emotional problem at home, school, or work. If this can be identified and eliminated, fine, but if not, and if the Stress Formula won't budge the pain, perhaps a hair analysis for minerals would help. (Poisoning from a heavy metal—lead, mercury, arsenic, or cadmium—frequently gives rise to muscle aches.)

Also try ice on a sore muscle; the shrinking effect will relieve the pain of an inflammation.

If the doctor tries a shot of cortisone and it helps, one didn't follow the Stress Program vigorously enough, because that program is designed to recharge the adrenals.

A Level II backache is the tightness you feel in the back or between the shoulder blades after standing all day or bending over a desk or sitting and typing for several hours. Pantothenic acid (200 to 300 mg) and calcium (1000 mg) at bedtime should allow child or adult to leap out of bed the next morning without a twinge.

A Level III backache lasts half the day and is associated with stiffness. A day in bed, pantothenic acid, calcium, and the Stress Formula should make it disappear. If this backache can be related to extra work, a long drive, too much exercise, or a visit from a not too welcome in-law, then okay: call it stress. But if it lasts too long and shoots down a leg or is associated with fever, some more specific diagnosis has to be made to prevent falling into Level IV.

X-rays must be done for a Level IV backache. The pain is constant, severe, forces the victim to bed, and requires codeine for suppression. No matter what the cause—disc, TB, fracture, congenital anomaly—the pain is a stress and the Stress Formula must be used along with whatever the doctor is doing.

In Level V, the patient is in the hospital under the care of a surgeon, who must do something soon, because this pain requires morphine. Nutritional supports must be continued in any case.

Brittle bones, or *osteogenesis imperfecta,* is the congenital condition of easy breakability of the bones. The collagen tissue is defective in amount or position, so the bones have no reinforcement (like the metal rods in concrete walks) and sometimes break as easily as chalk.

Parents of children with this condition tell us that stress, changing weather, different diets and nutrients all have an effect, but not consistently. A child may break several bones in a few weeks, then go a year with no trouble. There seems very little cause-and-effect relationship with anything, although stress will make these children worse.

A Level V child may have broken bones before birth and break his arms and legs in several places during delivery. A Level III child may break his upper arm when he pitches a fast ball at age seven; just the act of stopping his arm quickly will crack the bone. A Level II child will have a broken bone when hit directly, although the force did not seem great enough to do so.

Because the bones are involved, it makes sense to see that one to two grams of calcium are provided, along with vitamin D (500 to 1000 units per day) plus magnesium, phosphorus, and all the other minerals, and especially vitamin C, because of its known effect in aiding supportive tissues. Have big doses—5000 mg per day—ever been given to these children? Along with lots of B complex?

We know that bone-brittleness is a genetic problem, but genes make enzymes, and vitamins and minerals make enzymes work optimally. There has to be a reason why some children are but bags of broken bones while others are relatively well. Perhaps supernutrition might change the outlook.

Bursitis is an inflammation of a bursa, a condition rarely seen in children. A bursa is a flat space lined with mucus-secreting cells over which tendons and muscles glide. The shoulder tip is an area that commonly becomes inflamed; housemaid's knee is another example. The bursae get infected or inflamed and become tender, red, and swollen. The doctor may find calcium deposits therein, and he may want to give a cortisone shot. Because such a shot has a local effect (limited systemic effect) and because the condition is painful, perhaps you should let him go ahead. But the presence of the condition means that one must do something about the diet and the nutrients, especially by taking the Stress Formula.

A hair analysis might be a good idea if there is calcium in the bursa, since one should determine if the body is storing an overabundance in the soft tissues or if the calcium is coming out of the bones and depositing itself in areas of inflammation. Treatment would vary depending on stress, diet, activity level, and similar factors.

Cramps in the muscles of children are so common they are usually ignored or referred to as growing pains or shin splints. They are likely to occur after an active child has been asleep for an hour or two. He awakens screaming, clutching his shin, calf, instep, or thigh as if stabbed. It is a real spasm; you can feel the tight muscle fibers. Massage, hot towels, aspirin finally get him back to sleep. Spasms may recur nightly or monthly. Because they are more likely in the lower extremities following exercise, they are believed to be caused by accumulation of lactic acid or by the overutilization of calcium.

It is usually a simple matter to give extra calcium, upping the usual 1000 mg at bedtime (which also has a calming effect on the whole child). Some doctors also use magnesium to relax muscles. Vitamin D, 500 to 1000 units a day, might increase the absorption of calcium, but this tends to put the calcium into the bones. If the child is already on milk and some form of vitamin D and has these cramps, change to cod-liver oil and calcium tablets (or dolomite or bone meal). Sometimes stopping the milk will stop the cramps (which raises the question of allergy).

A B$_6$ deficiency is likely to explain finger and toe cramps. People who have these usually are older—not growing. They awaken in the middle of the night with aching feet that seem half asleep. Massaging them helps. This condition is better described as neuritis and it may be solved by 100 mg of B$_6$ nightly.

Uterine cramps (severe enough to put one to bed during menstrual periods) can be assuaged with calcium or dolomite tablets, but it takes a couple of weeks to get a priming dose in.

People who seem to overreact to intramuscular shots with pain that is incapacitating usually are low in calcium. A muscle low in calcium will cramp down harder and longer than a muscle properly supplied. ☐

If your child loves a food so much that he must eat it daily, it is probably bad for him.

Metabolize 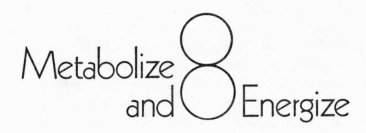 and Energize

Usually the stomach accepts what we send it. Like a good servant, it starts to work, does what it can, and then sends the food on to the intestines to be sorted out. The small bowel, twenty feet or so in length, is equipped to further break down plant and animal matter; it absorbs what it can and should, then dumps the unused portion into the large bowel for extraction of more water. A bowel movement is the residue. The digestive tube is no alchemist or magician; it cannot make human energy, human protein, or human bone if the raw materials are not put into it in the first place.

It is nonsense to believe we are supposed to get sick. Our bodies give us clues all the time that some biochemical pathway is being improperly nourished. Now that we are armed with science and experience, it is up to us to call a halt to this waste of our time and money and well-being.

If many babies can drink and sleep and laugh and grow without colic or diarrhea or vomiting or appendicitis, then ideally all should be able to do so. It is now well proved that the early mother-child interrelationship is all-important for the child's psychic and intellectual development later on. And it has been shown that the first milk (colostrum) from the mother is chock-full of important proteins and white cells which the baby must swallow to "seed" his intestinal immune system. All that is necessary is to feed the pregnant woman properly, give a little help during labor and delivery, and lovingly hand her baby to her right after delivery. She knows what to do and the baby knows what to do. Just leave them alone!

On the other hand, if a baby comes from a mother who has had a stressful or poorly nourished pregnancy, he will be likely to suffer milk allergy or other problems. The mother is exhausted; she may be unable to breast-feed the child, so she feeds him cow's milk. He might be able to survive drinking this milk, but the pasteurization, homogenization, and the addition of irradiated ergosterol (vitamin D) is just sufficient to make the muscles of the intestines cramp. He is colicky. He is placed on soybean milk, but he reacts to the corn syrup in the formula and gets gas and diarrhea. He gets pheno-barbitol to calm him down, and he reacts adversely and screams all night. The already tired parents are further stressed.

If this same child did not react intestinally, he might instead develop a respiratory allergy to milk—watery nose or attacks of asthma. The most common sequence is this: the mucus and swollen tissue in the nasal passages plug up the Eustachian tubes that run from the throat to the middle ear, infection follows (stress), and antibiotics are given (chemical stress); the child becomes susceptible to these infections and develops swollen adenoids and deafness (stress); by age two to three he has had tubes put in his eardrums and has had his adenoids removed (surgical stress). Now his adrenal glands are really exhausted and he develops asthma, insomnia, hyperactivity, skin rashes, hives, or bedwetting.   Stress leads to stress.

It should be clear that the place to halt this vicious cycle is at the beginning.   We were trained to believe that modified cow's milk was as good for babies as breast milk.   That grand experiment has been a failure.   The high incidence of intestinal and ear infection, allergies, hyperactivity, and—yes—even obesity and vascular problems can be related directly or indirectly to giving cow's milk to babies.   (If the first milk from the cow to the calf is pasteurized the calf won't drink it, or if it does, it dies within six weeks.)

I hope we can get the obstetricians to shoulder some of the blame.   Often their insistence on restrictive diets during pregnancy allows a woman to come to parturition so exhausted that nursing her equally indifferent baby is the last thing on her mind.   The movement toward natural feeding and away from artificial approaches is the best thing that could happen to mothers, babies, *and* harassed pediatricians.

The following intestinal problems can frequently be controlled or cured by a nutritional approach.   Do not however, wait while you test out these ideas.   Let your doctor know about anything that seems particularly troublesome and get definitive treatment.   Babies dehydrate rapidly and can suffer permanent harm or even die if they have a surgical problem that is progressing while you are trying to treat it with herb tea.

Anal fissure is an important clue that something intestinal is happening or has just happened.   Usually a large, firm, dry stool has passed and torn the skin at the anal opening. Once it is open, even a normal pasty stool will keep it raw and perhaps bleeding.   It's like trying to paint the roof when it's raining; you dab ointment on the area, but there really isn't time for it to rest and heal.

A Level II baby would show a minor crack. A dab of vitamin E oil, petroleum jelly, A and D ointment, or zinc oxide after each bowel movement should have it healed in three to six days. If it is a breast-fed baby, the mother must consider what she ate a day or two before the crack appeared (chocolate, citrus food, peaches, anything new or strange to her diet). If the crack was caused by a large, hard stool (which doesn't occur in babies that are breast-fed exclusively), then milk is the culprit. Once mothers were told to add corn syrup or molasses to loosen the movements. Now we are convinced that sugar (except lactose) in the diet should be avoided, so mixing prune juice, strained prunes, wheat germ, brewer's yeast, or some strained vegetables (do it yourself) with the milk is considered safer and more physiologically sound. (No mineral oil for young or old.) A milk change might be in order. A baby under six months of age who is continuously constipated should be changed to soybean milk or a meat formula.

In the next levels of anal fissure, much bleeding and sores all about the skin between the buttocks suggest a milk allergy and/or a secondary infection. The use of vitamin A (up to 25,000 units per day for a week or two by mouth), along with 20 to 50 mg of zinc given orally seems rational, assuming that there is something wrong with the healing ability of the skin. Be sure to stop using any vitamins with sugar, additives, or colors. Vitamin C (100 mg twice a day) helps healing. If the baby is over six to twelve months, the suggested foods in Chapter 2 would be best. (See also Afterword). Continue the above-mentioned ointments for the anal crack. Obvious broken-skin sores might heal faster if a little ointment containing polymyxin, bacitracin, or neomycin is used. The skin rapidly becomes sensitive to these, just as it does to any ointment with the suffix "caine," but a few germs will be killed.

The combination of sores, fissures, and loose, watery, stools (Level III or IV) in a bottle-fed baby almost always means an allergy. Goat's milk (best if fresh) is more constipating than soy milk usually, but any change in the diet takes twenty-four to forty-eight hours to be reflected in the stool frequency and consistency; wait that long for results—but not much longer. Excess gas would be a clue that the milk is fermenting and not being digested. Try a change to soy or meat formula or even a carbohydrate-free (CHO-Free) milk until you have found a satisfactory answer. If you haven't already done so, now would be the time to add acidophilus culture orally to see if a proper type of bacteria could replace the ill-suited one; this can be done any time a baby's stools smell putrid, fetid, or like some adults'. (*See* Colic, below.)

On several occasions I have been able to clear up these unhappy, messy babies with a B complex shot. The effects on the stools, the skin, and the irritability are almost miraculous in just twenty-four to forty-eight hours. I am assuming that the B vitamins have done two things: (1) improved the functioning of the enzymes in the lining cells of the intestines that split the fats, carbohydrates, and proteins into nonallergic, digestible units; and (2) added some nourishment to the adrenal glands so they can produce cortisone to help control the allergy (in the skin and intestines).

All these serious things could follow an anal fissure. The fissure is only a clue that tells us that the baby has the potential of slipping all the way down to Level IV. It doesn't always happen, but a little remedial action early is good insurance against future grief. (*See* Colic, Constipation, Diarrhea, later in this chapter.)

Anorexia is loss of appetite. When it appears suddenly it frightens parents, since they feel, often justifiably, that the child is about to become sick. Most children show fluctuations in appetite from time to time and, provided they are otherwise active and cheerful, the fluctuations mean nothing that I know of.

But a Level II anorectic child would ask to be put to bed

or would fall asleep on the floor at odd times, or he'd become crabby or stumble or look pale. Something is invading his system; despite his protests, some action must be taken. A fever is a clear indication. Vitamin C is the first line of defense—don't wait until the disease is diagnosable. A stress allowed the invasion, and the invasion has escalated the stress. Vitamin C is a general, all-purpose anti-infective agent, so it might work on a germ or a virus or an allergy. According to Dr. Linus Pauling and others, the more that is given and the sooner, the better for the patient.

Try the following:

- Infants, one to eight months—100 mg of vitamin C every hour for twenty-four hours, then every two hours if things are better or are tapering off. (One teaspoon of vitamin C powder contains 2.5 grams of vitamin C. Dissolve one teaspoon in 3 ounces or so of water. A little honey—tupelo, preferably—might help it go down. A teaspoon of this every hour or so should supply the 100 mg.)
- Children, eight months to five years—increase the dose to 200 to 250 mg by making the solution twice as strong. Mix it with juice, freeze it, and call it a popsicle if you must, but get it down.
- Older children, when able to swallow tablets—give 500 to 1000 mg every hour or two; use time-release capsules, if available. (Many adults take 1000 or more mg every hour or two if they feel they are coming down with something.)

Eighty-five percent of children's infections are due to the "virus that is going around." The fever lasts seventy-two hours and the cough or the diarrhea that follows usually for seven days. The vitamin C treatment is not guaranteed to stop the illness, but if the fever lasts only one day and the other symptoms only three days, the child is 50 percent ahead.

If, however, you did not treat the disease in time, or if

it was too tough for the treatment, ـe child has slipped into Level III. He has a fever above 102 or 103 degrees that does not respond to aspirin (one grain of aspirin for each ten pounds of weight) and a comfortable, hot bath. Or he has a febrile convulsion, or he gets stiff and nonresponsive. Or he is vomiting and dehydrated or is coughing, wheezing, and turning blue. Don't wait. Get him to the doctor or the emergency room.

If it is found that he has meningitis, pneumonia, or a kidney infection, he is in Level V. Antibiotics work beautifully for these infections, and little residual damage from the disease will be noted—*if* you (and we) act in time.

The fact that you pretreated him at home with the vitamin C and have nourished him well all his life will mean that his time in the hospital will be brief. Your job is to oversee his medication and his diet. You can't rely on hospital food. You must check the labels on the intravenous bottle and suggest amino acids instead of glucose. And you must remind the doctor that vitamin C should be continued in huge doses— probably better if given intravenously. The B complex, especially B_6 (100-mg dosages), is valuable. Calcium will make him comfortable and will help the C work. Be pleasant but firm. Most hospitals discourage parent participation in the therapy, but this is your child under stress. Even if they think you are a nut, smile and nod your head, but be firm.

Anorexia of the two- to three-year-old appears almost on the day of the second birthday. And that's not all. He begins to whine. He may be cutting his three-year molars and practicing for adolescent noncompliance by not wanting to use the toilet. Even a Level I child has some of these characteristics, but because he is basically so cheerful and has been eating properly all along, his parents don't have to worry.

The stress of being two to three years of age may be felt more keenly by the parents than by the child. As the mother usually knows, if he would just eat he would feel better, and if he felt better he would eat. One of the chief jobs of the pediatrician is to offer reassurance at the two-year-old checkup: "Remember now, he won't eat for a year. He will gain only about two to four pounds this next year, so he will eat in a year what he did in a month when he was three months old." Sometimes this helps to keep the parents from fighting at mealtime.

Most of these children do better if allowed to nibble— six small feedings spread out during the day. The rule is: If he can get up and walk around, he is probably getting enough calories. However, it is very important that these calories be nutritious ones. There should be no sugar in the house; if he tastes sweets, he'll want nothing else. "Naked" carbohydrates starve the enzyme systems that normally metabolize the calories. If allowed such foods he will develop a deficiency. Then he will get sick (stress) and won't eat. He will become further depleted. Parents and grandparents worry that he must eat something, so they give him cookies, puddings, boxed cereals, pop, and the like—antinutrients. He cuts teeth (a stress) and fades a little more. He has learned that he can get attention by going hungry.

He is down into Level III by now. The doctor checks his blood for anemia, almost hoping he can find something to get this family to relax. He suggests a trial of no milk and an iron tonic. This may help the Level II or III child, whose parents by now feel they have done everything and are turning their attention to other things. The child is not getting emotional fortification and so he outgrows the problem.

Level IV must be the child who has been through all the above and feels miserable unless he eats sweets. He is often surly, angry, still has temper tantrums, won't go to bed, won't be trained, won't cuddle—a real monster. He has slipped almost imperceptibly into a biochemical bind. There may be no skin, nail, or tongue clues to give away the deficiencies.

No one can predict when the child is eighteen months old if he is going to be anorectic a year later. Assume that he could be. All those under two should be treated the same way, because once they hit twenty-four to thirty months, treatment by nourishment is just this side of impossible.

Do what you can early, but try this if he has already hit Level IV anorexia:

Cod-liver oil drops sufficient to give 400 units or so of vitamin D and 5000 to 10,000 units of vitamin A. If he won't eat liver or carrots or other good sources of vitamin A, this amount might be increased temporarily.

Vitamin C, especially if the child is infection-prone and is upset when he cuts teeth (a stress): 100 mg minimum, and up to 500 mg every hour or two if he is showing the behavioral signs of anorexia.

Vitamin B complex is a well-known appetite stimulant, but its evil taste precludes easy administration. (You should have started this way back at seven to ten months to teach him that all good food is not sweet.) Some will open up a capsule of B complex and mix the contents in cereal, honey, home-made peanut butter, or juice. Begin with small amounts and try to build up to at least one to three teaspoons of brewer's yeast a day or at least 10 to 20 mg of each of the Bs per day. Wheat germ sprinkled on whole-grain cereal or toast may work. If he is anemic because he has been drinking a lot of milk, an iron and B complex vitamin may be just the ticket.

Dolomite powder tastes like chalk and has calcium and magnesium in it. If the child is off milk, aim for one gram of calcium per day and 500 mg of magnesium per day. Try mixing it with tortillas the way some Mexicans do (though they get it naturally from grinding their meal in limestone mortars).

Vegetable oil is necessary—at least one to two teaspoons per day.

You don't want him to eat a lot; you only want him to

eat enough so he will grow properly, have good teeth and bones, and be cheerful more than half the time. No desserts except fruit. Small amounts on his plate: one tablespoon of fish or chicken, seven peas (raw or slightly cooked), and a quarter of a piece of whole-wheat bread buttered is a big meal for the average two- to three-year-old. Let him nibble. Feed him a little supper early, so his blood sugar won't be so low when the family eats.

But what happens if you've done all this, or have done what you can, and he is still a reluctant diner? Some research indicates that he may need zinc. Zinc is necessary for the optimum functioning of the taste buds. (Adults with severe zinc deficiencies say that most foods have a putrid taste.) Assuming he is deficient and the daily requirement is 15 mg, try to get 50 to 100 mg of zinc chelate into him daily for a month or in addition to the other nutrients. Then try to feed him the foods high in zinc. Whole grains, nuts and seeds are good.

According to some parents, the behavior and appetites of their two- to three-year-olds are so intolerable and the children so full of food allergies that they surely qualify for Level V classification. Such kids eat only white bread, sugar, and cookies and drink pop. Usually they have circles under their eyes, suffer hay fever or asthma, are frequently hyperactive Jekyll-and-Hyde types. They are allergic to milk (at least pasteurized-homogenized milk), eggs, peanuts, citrus foods, corn. Pancakes with syrup, boxed cereal, apple juice, and McDonald's hamburgers seem to be it. The parents try the starvation technique to motivate their child to eat, and after three days of starvation, they can't stand seeing him shrivel up, so they go out for a Big Mac. No way are they able to get any tonic or vitamins into this stone of a kid.

I have been delighted to find that a shot or two of B complex vitamins in the hip muscle is often enough to reverse the whole picture. The child sleeps better, feels better, and eats better; we have broken the vicious cycle.   His noneating had caused a B-vitamin deficiency plus adrenal-gland exhaustion that prevented his brain from getting messages from his appetite center.   The low blood sugar level also prevented his neocortex from perceiving the proper environmental messages. The shot of B vitamins may have turned on his intestinal digestive enzymes, allowing him to enjoy the food presented.

These children usually come from mothers who had a stressful pregnancy.   The congenital poor functioning of the adrenals allows food allergies to appear and the child is suspicious of everything except sugar.   I feel that all this time-consuming, frustrating problem could have been avoided if the mother had been nourished properly during pregnancy and if she had breast-fed this child and begun giving him nourishing food early.

If all the above measures haven't worked, a hair analysis for mineral imbalance and heavy-metal poisonings (especially lead) would be the next step.

Anorexia nervosa is usually the diagnosis for the young pubescent (usually a girl) who stops eating.   Just like that, she refuses.   At a time when most adolescents are wolfing down everything in sight, she adamantly refuses to ingest more than three bites a day plus maybe six ounces of water.   "I don't know" is her stock answer.   She may be successful in school; her home is no better or worse in the amount and quality of emotional supports than others; she has friends, but she won't eat even for them.

Psychiatrists have found that for a variety of reasons these girls don't want to accept adult womanhood with all the responsibilities it entails.   "If I don't eat I won't grow.   If I don't grow, I won't become a woman" seems to be the Alice-in-Wonderland paralogic underlying their refusal to eat.   Fear of fat explains some cases.   During psychotherapy they are frequently hospitalized, and by the use of a behavior-modification approach (they are not permitted to go home or have TV or some other "fun" things) some food is gotten into their stomachs, at least enough to maintain a predetermined weight.

There are few other conditions in which psychiatry and biochemistry dovetail so closely as in this. We know enough about nutrition to know that in times of stress (in this case, early adolescence and starvation) the body needs more nutriment rather than less. Depletion could easily alter anyone's perception of herself and the world to the point that a new and greater stress is added to the first. When the brain is depleted of vitamins and nutrients it cannot handle even the most supportive stimuli from the environment; it sees only threats or problems. Trusted friends and family find they are talking to an unresponsive animal, not to the child's cortex, where she used to "live."

If nutritional supports have been followed from the beginning, a girl should be less vulnerable to the stresses of these years, which include pubescence, rapid growth, peer-group and academic pressures, and unresolved domestic forces.

There are few clues to warn parents about anorexia nervosa, and a secure Level I girl could drop all the way to Level V in no time. It is rare, but be forewarned. As soon as the growth starts to spurt and breasts begin to bud, up all the nutrients, check out the diet, and look her in the eyes once in a while and ask "How are you doing? Are you okay?" This is the minimum we can do for our children.

Appendicitis is a surgical condition; an inflammation of the wormlike outpouching of the cecum can kill a healthy person in forty-eight hours. Genetic factors are strongly suggested. I know a set of twins who had appendicitis within six months of each other. I remember a calm mother calling me one day with the following information: "I had my appendix out when I was eleven. Two of my girls had appendectomies when they were ten. Now my last daughter, who is nine and a half, has a temperature of a hundred one and a constant pain and tenderness in the lower right side of her abdomen which feels worse when she jumps up and down. What do you think?"

"What's the white blood count?" I responded smartly. What she needed, of course, was the name of a surgeon. And the surgeon hardly needed the blood count, since the story was classic. The girl had appendicitis and surgery was carried out in the routine manner.

As with so many conditions in the human body, environmental factors will allow a genetic problem to become manifest as a diagnosable disease. Appendicitis is almost unknown among people who live on a "primitive" diet (no sugar, white flour, or low-fiber foods). This fact gives you one more reason never to allow antinutrients or processed foods into the house or the mouths of your family. If you know that the trait is in the family, you can bring that up when your children tire of raw vegetables, whole-wheat bread, nuts, fruits, and salads and ask you "When are we going to have something good?" Tell them "I would love to give you junk, but I'm afraid you might die of appendicitis, like Aunt Ellie." That might work for twenty minutes.

A tip: The *pain of gas* or intestinal flu is usually around the navel and comes and goes; a big loose stool should provide temporary relief and the abdomen should be doughy albeit queasy, not tender in any one consistent area. The *pain of appendicitis* is usually in the right lower area of the abdomen and doesn't go away with the passage of gas or stool; it feels like the worst gas pain you have ever had, and it gets worse if you jump up and down.

Don't fool around if your child has stomach pain that

stays. It is all right to give vitamin C, because pain is a stress, but give it on the *way* to the hospital, not *instead* of going.

If there is a genetic tendency to appendicitis, it is especially important for someone of authority in the family to monitor bowel movements occasionally (without appearing odd) to make sure none of your children is having firm, dry, pellets instead of rather sloppy, or at least pasty, eliminations.

Because the disease is a stress and the surgery is a further stress, get the basic vitamins plus the Stress Formula started while the victim is still in the hospital. Extra vitamin A (50,000 units per day) and zinc chelate (100 mg per day) for two weeks should help healing. Rub a little vitamin E oil on the wound daily; it might keep the scarring to a minimum.

Celiac disease is characterized by the passage of two to six large, foul-smelling, greasy bowel movements a day. It is accompanied by wasted buttocks and a large, protuberant, bloated abdomen and occasionally, if chronic and severe, by slow growth. It is now known to be due to a specific inability of the intestinal and pancreatic enzymes to digest and absorb gluten, the protein fraction of wheat and some other grains.

A food allergy to other proteins can mimic the problem; milk, eggs, beef, legumes, nuts, could all do this, but never as severely or with such devastation to the whole body as allergy to wheat gluten. Wheat flour is in so many things, and it takes only a small amount to put the bowels out of whack for one to two weeks.

Almost everyone—except Level I, perfect people—has a big, sloppy, loose bowel movement every once in a while ("something I ate") or cramps and diarrhea for a day ("the one-day flu"), but with celiac disease this goes on and on. (*See* Diarrhea, below.) Once it starts following the flu or a stress it seems to perpetuate itself because the first few days of flu have also sloughed off most of the lining cells of the intestines wherein lie the enzymes that split the food particles into absorbable simple sugars, amino acids, and fats. So even if the victim stops wheat and everything else that is suspect, the condition remains until the cells mature again and become functional enzyme-producers. These cells need nutrients to regrow and refunction, but they cannot refunction unless they are renourished, and they cannot be renourished unless they refunction—a Catch-22 situation.

A Level II problem drops into a Level IV or V in about two to four days. Time will correct the condition in a healthy youngster, but to ease the suffering and waste and debility we try water and a few minerals by mouth and a few vitamin B injections in the muscle to circumvent the natural oral routine that is not functioning. Usually in forty-eight hours the patient is constipated; the vitamin Bs have gone to the cells via the reliable blood supply and put them together.

If celiac disease is the problem, try to stay away from wheat; but one may find the attacks are less serious or prolonged with the daily ingestion of lots of the B complex and brewer's yeast (50 to 100 mg of each per day; no wheat germ). Because stress is usually the inciting agent, if the wheat intake has been constant or nil, use the Stress Formula. Pancreatic granules should work, but they may not.

Colic is not serious unless you are the parents of the suffering baby. A Level II baby might have it once a week if his nursing mother ate onions or cabbage. He might be bloated and bent and crying for six to twenty-four hours while the offender moves from stomach to rectum where he can pass the fermented products. Not much need be done, although rocking, a suppository, some herb tea (comfrey is one), and a solution of potassium might give temporary relief.

A Level III baby would have a daily attack usually between 5:00 and 10:00 P.M., when supper is being prepared or eaten or when father or mother come home or when the family is trying to watch their favorite TV show. The child appears to be hungry and usually gets fed, but seems to cry more or throw everything up.

Tapping the abdomen with finger, as if testing a melon, usually gives the message that the intestines are "ripe" with gas, so a small enema (an ounce of body temperature tap water injected with a syringe into the rectum) is tried with indifferent results. The somewhat surprised baby may squirt out the water with some gas and stool, but the problem is that the gas is entrapped in the twenty or so feet of bowel from the stomach on down, and you might have unloaded only the last foot of the colon and rectum.

Something must be done to prevent the gas from forming or to prevent this particular baby from being so aware of the gas he thinks it is a bayonet attack. Even Level I babies have some gas, but they ignore it or think it is fun. There are probably at least three organs in this baby that are not functioning optimally: (1) the brain, which seems to have a low threshold for noticing incoming stimuli; (2) the intestinal tract, which doesn't seem to be digesting the milk properly, with the result that it ferments, producing more gas than the baby can handle; and (3) the adrenal glands, which help to alleviate allergies with cortisone and apparently are not fulfilling their job.

1. The limbic system of the brain is at least partially responsible for filtering out incoming messages from the external environment as well as those from the body itself. (See Chapter 9.) This system is a network of nerves that secretes norepinephrine predominantly; if the enzymes do not produce norepinephrine, it is assumed that too many messages will get through to the cortex, the perceiving area of the brain. The cortex can only conclude from this sensory overload that there is a stress, and it will in turn send an emergency signal to the pituitary gland, which will alert the adrenal glands to produce cortisone and adrenalin preparing the body for flight or fight.

One approach for the colicky baby, then, is to strengthen the filtering chemicals of the limbic system. By providing B vitamins we help the enzyme to make norepinephrine. B_1, B_2, B_3, and B_6 in amounts of 10 to 50 mg per day for a few days might be helpful.

2. The intestinal tract is lined with cells containing enzymes that are supposed to split the carbohydrates, fats, and proteins into their simple forms to be absorbed. The same B vitamins should help these enzymes also. The gas may be due to the fermentation of foods by unfriendly bacteria. To try to replace the smelly, putrefactive bacteria with the more physiological bacteria that give breast-fed babies' stools that yeasty, "bread baking in the oven" smell, use only lactose as the carbohydrate in artificial milk and give some lactobacillus orally three or four times a day. Some nutritionists supplement the diet with pancreatic enzymes to promote this digestive action, but these enzymes can cause a nasty rash around the anus.

In colic, the muscular outer layer of the intestine is cramping up on the contained gas, so quieting this action should ease the pain, especially if the stools are loose and greenish (that's bile coming through so fast it doesn't have a chance to change color). Dolomite powder should help—up to one-half to one gram a day divided into small frequent doses, with perhaps the main amount in midafternoon just before the bad time. Bone meal or calcium powder (or solution) would be alternatives. Calcium and magnesium also have a calming action on the nervous system. Potassium has an effect on muscles and may be valuable.

The loose green stools might have blood in them, so don't forget the vitamin C. If, when changing the diapers for the umpteenth time, you see some sores and anal fissure or much redness about the anus, an allergy is a likely factor (see Anal Fissure, above).

3. The adrenal glands would certainly have become ex-

hausted from the stress of pain and crying over a period of days. If they become depleted, an allergy approach could be worthwhile. Wait a few days before changing milks, if possible, then if the adrenals need help, add B_6 and pantothenic acid (grind up the pills—100 to 200 mg a day) for a while. The body is believed to have more cortisone in the 6:00-to-8:00 A.M. period than in the evening; evening colic may be a reflection of this low level of circulating cortisone (really cortisol).

The most likely candidates for colic and/or milk allergy are babies born of mothers who had a stressful (perhaps unwanted) pregnancy, had allergies themselves, had a difficult delivery, or delivered their babies prematurely. It is possible that the baby's adrenal glands suffered along with the mother's, and indeed may have been partially supplying her body, so at birth he was operating with a relative deficiency or exhausted adrenals. For a number of reasons, these babies are frequently not breast-fed; too bad, since these are the very babies most likely to suffer on a diet of bottle milk. If a baby is born from a suboptimal pregnancy or delivery, it makes some sense to give the Stress Formula prophylactically.

Level IV colic is seen in babies who cry all the time. (I am sure that some of these are in danger of becoming battered children.) By now the milk has been changed several times, all the above nutritional tricks have been tried, and the harassed parents just want some relief. It is not a dirty trick or sign of weakness to place the baby in the hospital for a few days if a grandmother is nervous about taking the responsibility. By the time the baby gets to Level IV a vicious cycle often has started up. The baby started the problem, sure, but the parents can unwittingly continue it by their handling. It must be embarrassing for them to call the hospital the next day and learn that the baby slept peacefully all night.

The old standard prescription was to give some barbiturate (such as phenobarbital), which is safe and occasionally works. Rule: If phenobarbital makes the baby worse, he is probably hyperactive, since phenobarbital dopes the cortex and does nothing for the limbic system. Benadryl and Phenergan are basically antihistaminics with a sedative side effect. Rule: If these are beneficial, an allergy is the likely cause. Drugs related to belladonna suppress the intestinal cramping; if they work, calcium might be helpful.

The treatment that I have been delighted with and wish I had known about twenty-five years ago is the injection of the B vitamins into the baby's muscle. It must help the limbic system, the intestines directly, and the adrenal glands. Just .2 to .3 cc intramuscularly will quiet the most colicky baby overnight—well, maybe 80 percent of them. The 20 percent who are not improved, or who get even worse temporarily, are histamine releasers and are usually then helped with calcium and magnesium (for example, dolomite).

Level V babies are an enigma to most of us, and we usually just snow them with a long list of drugs. I worry about these babies and try to be as supportive and sympathetic with the parents as possible. A fresh look might uncover a urinary problem, a partial bowel obstruction, a brain injury, a domestic psychiatric imbalance—anything. Usually, however, a serious problem precludes normal growth, and colicky babies almost always grow rapidly. They usually think the pain is hunger, and to solve that they eat.

Constipation is the passage of hard, dry (large or small) stools; the frequency is not important. The hard, dry consistency is the sole determining factor.

Breast-fed babies are hardly ever constipated; there must have been a few over the centuries, of course, but it is very rare. It's amazing how these babies may have a bowel movement infrequently and yet it is so liquid. Sometimes a week will go by and the worried parents think maybe he is obstructed, but he is happy, vigorous, sucks and swallows well, his urine is plentiful, and he does not vomit. If you can't stand it one more minute, you might poke the end of a lubricated finger, a suppository, or a sliver of soap into the rectum, especially if he seems to look a little bloated. You will probably be rewarded with a cupful or so of golden, yeasty- or acid-smelling fluid. Occasionally it may be chartreuse in color, but a Level I baby should not have any green or frothy stools. That would get him to Level II.

When cow's milk or solid food (especially rice, apple-sauce, or bananas) is added (this can begin at six to eight months) the stools may begin to have firmness and become malodorous.

Some babies, children, and adults seem prone to consti-pation, and chronic constipation is now believed to be a causa-tive factor in appendicitis, diverticulosis, hemorrhoids, anal fissures and ulcers, and varicose veins. The chief argument of those who hold that diet is the culprit is that these conditions are virtually nonexistent in people who eat a natural, "Stone-Age" diet. The offenders in the modern diet are sugar, white-flour products, packaged foods, pasteurized-homogenized milk, polished rice—processed foods in general. It is a shame that so many people believe they have to rely on laxatives for nor-mal bowel movements.

The best products for alleviating hard, dry, stools are bulk, moisture holders, or softeners. And this is just what Mother Nature offers us. Almost every food in a natural state contains the proper amount of roughage for that particular food (raw vegetables, most fruits, seeds, and nuts, for exam-ple). Bananas are considered constipating and prunes may make one's movement a little sloppy (see Anal Fissure, above).

The two- to three-year-old tends to become constipated if he is still consuming large amounts of milk, if he has been allowed to eat crackers and sugar products, and if his appetite

falls off—as it is apt to do. He may go from Level II constipation right down to Level IV (someone may have to dig it
out) in one short week. This is why it is so important that the
infant get some kind of roughage—a little brewer's yeast or
wheat germ or desiccated liver powder or bran—almost every
day from six to eight months so that these food supplements
will not come as a big surprise later on. Cooked vegetables
for the infant would be changed to steamed or just barely
cooked for the toddler with four molars. Then mainly raw
vegetables, including a daily salad, for the over-three-year-old
who has cut all his baby teeth (twenty). The same rule would
apply to nuts, seeds, and fruits. The whole fruit or vegetable
is better for teeth, gums, and nutrition than the juice alone.

Primitive diets pass from mouth to rectum in less than a
day. The average "civilized" diet slows this to two days or
more. The prolonged reabsorption of water causes constipation, and there is increased putrefaction from the activity of
bacteria (*see* Bad breath, Chapter 5). There is some evidence
that prolonged constipation in a susceptible person could lead
to cancer of the lower bowel, because a byproduct of cholic
acid (in bile) changes to a carcinogen when stool passage is
delayed.

It is much easier to be preventive than to be therapeutic.
Begin the infant with breast milk, add only natural foods when
solids are introduced, use some roughage daily for a lifetime.
If you find you are reading books in the bathroom, there
may be something wrong with your intestinal peristalsis; don't
call the doctor (unless you are temporarily in Level V)—call
your greengrocer.

Cramps (abdominal) severe enough to come to the attention of the sufferer can be caused by gas. They usually occur
at the navel area, and come and go in cycles lasting a few
minutes. A Level I person stops, grimaces a little, and then

in a few seconds resumes his play or work. His cramps will be relieved by time, a loose bowel movement, or vomiting (often of the preceding two meals).

Level II cramps are usually the result of a food allergy, too much gas-forming food, or certain medicines. Sometimes a poorly functioning limbic system allows the child to be aware of the normal digestive process, and the Level II person responds by becoming crampy. An instance of this is the psychosomatic Monday-morning-before-school "I don't feel good" complaint, the culmination of such factors as low blood sugar, attempting too much over the weekend, eating junk foods, "forgetting" to have a bowel movement, and the thought of boring school. Nor is it just the poor student who suffers thus; it is often the conscientious one whose psyche drives him to high standards of achievement.

It is not easy for parents to know if this is a real sickness requiring the attentions of the doctor (Level IV or V), or if it should be handled with behavior-modification techniques (don't reward the child for having the stomachache and it will disappear). Many parents have sent their children to school half sick, thinking "I'm sure it's not serious." At about nine-thirty the teacher calls asking why you did not keep your sick child home, as she just threw up all over the classroom.

"I didn't know."

"She says she told you."

"Sorry."

How *do* you know? The doctor can give an opinion on whether the child has slipped into a IV or V level based on the child's history, palpation of the abdomen, and blood tests; his consultation would be worthwhile if you are unsure of yourself. Your aim is not to discipline the child because he does not have an organic disease but to try to determine why his cortex perceives a stomach problem. He is hanging in limbo somewhere between exaggerated normal function and an organic, diagnosable disease—a psychosomatic or somatopsychic tilt. This used to be called neurasthenia. *Hypochondriasis* is a label doctors still use when they cannot explain the physiology of the symptoms. It is into this rather uncharted wilderness we now venture. And nutrition can be the key.

The severity and chronicity of the cramps would determine whether a child or adult is in Level II or Level III, but the reasons for being on either level may be similar: perhaps just his individual sensitivity or awareness makes the symptoms more vivid for him and pushes him down to the lower level. Remember, you cannot live inside his body and perceive what he perceives; he is as unique as a snowflake. But we know he is not in Level I. The following suggestions hold for the sufferer from three years old well into adulthood.

1. Past history is helpful. If he was a colicky baby, a milk allergy and stress could combine to make him miserable. Therapy: stop dairy products for at least a month, use the Prevention Diet and vitamins. (*See* Tension-fatigue syndrome, Chapter 5.)

2. If he had much sickness as a baby (ear infections, colds, croup, bronchitis, intestinal flu, for example), he may have a chronic low-grade infection in the lymph glands of his abdomen (mesenteric adenitis). Therapy: Prevention Diet and vitamins with special emphasis on vitamin C, perhaps 1000 mg per day for a month. Sometimes the glands in the front and back of the neck are enlarged as a dubious clue, and their size would tell a parent how the therapy was going. An antibiotic for two weeks may be a godsend for these sickly ones, even though there are few clues that an infection is going on.

3. If the child is somewhat hyperactive and has emotion instability (Jekyll-and-Hyde mood swings), his vague

aches may arise from his sensitivity to all stimuli (just normal digestion is uncomfortable) and from his idiosyncratic response to fluctuating blood sugar (*see* Hypoglycemia, Chapter 9).

4. Pinworms, lead poisoning, anemia, constipation all must be considered.

5. A history of migraine or epilepsy in the family would suggest the possibility of some problem in the nervous system, for which the diagnosis of a specialist would be needed.

6. If the child's mother had a stressful pregnancy, this may be significant.

7. If a child has dark circles under his eyes, is snorting or zonking and is pale, think of allergy, especially milk. (*See* Tension-fatigue syndrome, Chapter 5.)

8. If he is terribly ticklish (goosey, sensitive), he could be having trouble with his limbic system (*see* Chapter 9). Therapy with the B vitamins and dolomite may be helpful.

Laboratory tests may be revealing. If there is a bacterial infection, the white blood count usually rises. (*See* Appendicitis, above.) Intestinal flu is a virus and is accompanied by a low or normal white blood count. A urinalysis may show pus, suggesting a bladder or kidney infection—which would be surprising since cramps usually are not associated with this infection, whose victims usually have burning on urination. Blood sedimentation rate may help to tell about strange, hidden, chronic infection (such as ileitis, nephritis, rheumatic fever). Many of these conditions can be improved with better nutrition, but you will need a doctor to monitor the course of the infection.

Cystitis is a bladder infection more common in girls than in boys. It is usually due to the E. coli bacteria, which is thought to cause the infection by moving from the rectal area to the vaginal area and thence up the shorter urethra to the bladder. This opportunist type of infection doesn't happen to all girls, so if they continue to acquire it, we should look for an obstruction or an anomaly that allows for stagnation.

If no tubing problem is obvious by x-ray or cystoscopy, then keeping the urine acidic seems sensible. Cranberry juice has been recommended, but the sugar that is added for palatability negates its effectiveness. Vitamin C is the safe acidifier, and 100 to 1000 mg per day is very safe; it might be continued for a lifetime. An occasional litmus test of the urine to monitor the acidity is the minimum care needed. Bacteria have trouble growing in acid urine. Get rid of the infection with antibiotics or sulfa drugs; if there is no structural problem, the vitamin C program should work.

If a boy gets cystitis, a full-scale test series is mandatory, because it suggests a serious obstructive problem.

Diabetes is a malfunction of the mechanism for carbohydrate utilization. It is not merely a lack of insulin from pancreas beta-cell atrophy. It may be that the whole pancreas, including digestive enzyme function, is exhausted. Some diabetics have a normal amount of insulin, but this hormone may not be active, or the cells that are supposed to turn glucose into glycogen do not respond to the insulin because of acidosis or inadequate B complex vitamin intake. Thyroid function also may play a role.

Some patients respond to the ingestion of certain foods (not just sugar or carbohydrates) with a sharp rise in blood glucose, an inappropriate response. This may be accompanied by physical or mental symptoms thought to be due to acidosis. If acidosis, it sometimes can be relieved by taking Golden Alka-Seltzer. Paradoxically, some find that a smaller intake of the same offender will relieve the symptoms. This response is the clue to the allergic-addictive syndrome (if one loves a food and must consume it daily, it suggests that *that* food is the cause of the symptoms).

Thus, some diabetes may be an allergic response to certain commonly eaten foods, or an autoimmune response to certain commonly eaten foods, or an autoimmune disease that prevents the full use of insulin.

In any event, an option is suggested. Big (stress) doses of vitamin C and the B complex, and the like (see Stress Formula) may alter the course. A period of fasting with careful monitoring of the blood sugar may reveal the true nature of the disease. Brewer's yeast is supposed to contain a glucose tolerance factor (B complex and chromium) and some diabetics have been able to reduce their insulin dose when taking three tablespoons of this a day.

Diarrhea is the passage of liquid stools, usually accompanied by cramps and gaseous explosiveness. The frequency of passage is above normal; some victims find it necessary to stay within a few feet of the toilet facilities to prevent an embarrassing leak. The condition is common; even a Level I baby, child, or adult is not immune, but his suffering is not severe and is soon over. He might call it the "one-day flu" and relate it to stress or bad piece of ham. An attack once every two or three years would be his rate. Breast-fed babies rarely have infectious diarrhea.

The Level II person might get diarrhea once a year and the routine would be as in intestinal flu: a day of vomiting and seven days (count 'em) days of diarrhea. He could be operating at a better level, so he should be sure to follow the basic diet and vitamins, and when he has experienced or knows he will experience a stress, he should take the Stress Formula prophylactically.

Level III people would have to run to the toilet on the first day of school, on their wedding day, or whenever faced with some new situation. It would appear that there is a direct connection between their brains and their intestines. In addition to the Prevention Diet and vitamin supplements, they would need to use the Stress Formula daily. They should experiment with possible food allergies and perhaps eliminate milk, coffee, eggs, corn, wheat, beef, and potatoes to see if some diet stress is keeping them on the brink of trouble.

In Level IV celiac disease and other causes of chronic diarrhea problems (malabsorption, short intestine, Crohn's disease, ulcerative colitis, ileitis, severe food allergy) might have to be diagnosed by the doctor with laboratory tests, x-rays, and a proctoscopic examination.

A more common Level IV baby, child, or adult might have been a Level II type until he came down with an attack of what seemed to be intestinal flu, but it kept on and on, well beyond the usual seven-day limit. Three possible diagnoses would now have to be considered: (1) The stress of the flu allowed a food allergy (usually milk or wheat) to appear. This is frequently seen in a baby, six to twelve months of age, who was recently weaned to the bottle and who falls ill with the flu that was circulating in the family. Because the others have had it before, they are somewhat immune and revive in a day or so, but the distress goes on and on until someone thinks of trying no milk at all. (2) A child gets the flu followed by diarrhea; it doesn't stop and is still slopping on after weeks. All the tests are negative, there are no bad bacteria cultured from a stool specimen, and the doctor calls it "chronic non-specific diarrhea." Sometimes a sulfa drug will help, for it appears that a variant of E. coli, the usual intestinal bacteria, has changed into something pathogenic. The parents usually have to put up with three to five big messes a day, and they try to find a diet of nutritious food they can sneak into the top end of this touchy tube that won't aggravate the lower end. Allowables may include rice, applesauce, a little chicken or lamb, some soy milk, and a bit of carrot. (3) A nasty bug has been picked up, perhaps salmonella (usually some fever and a rotten-egg smell to the stools give this away) or shigella, which causes the terrible chills, fever, and bloody diarrhea of dysentery. The former is not supposed to be treated with an antibiotic, since this may prolong the disease and could lead to a carrier state. The latter requires hospitalization and treatment with intravenous fluid and antibiotics.

The problem with diarrhea is that it is self-perpetuating as in the above three situations. It is assumed that the cells lining the length of the small bowel have been eroded and are functionally nonoperative. It seems prudent, if normal stool activity does not appear in two or three days, to try an injection or two of the B complex vitamins—no matter what the diagnosis is or what the doctor has outlined as treatment. It just might shorten the course of the illness.

Encopresis is the passing of some stool into the underclothing long after the child has been toilet-trained for bowel movements. It is usually considered a psychiatric problem, a form of passive aggression. The child, usually a boy, feels that he is being put down somehow, and he becomes depressed and resentful. Because he is unable to speak out (be orally aggressive), he becomes anally aggressive and lets a little bit of stool leak out to show the world and his parents what he thinks of them ("Poop on you!").

This problem cannot be ignored in the hope that it will disappear. The child smells bad and gets a rash; everyone else gets disgusted. The child seems to be indifferent to the problem, and indeed seems surprised when he finds the dollop of stool there. It is hard for his parents to believe that he is unaware of what has happened, since most adults are acutely sensitive to anything passing in this area.

Although psychiatric problems may produce this frustrating behavior, it is now felt that a variety of physiological imbalances get the "habit" started and that the attention gained thereby, although negative, becomes the reinforcer.

Sometimes the situation starts with the parents' efforts to toilet-train the child too early. The child develops a "holding pattern"; he feels that if this stuff is so important, it's probably smart to hang on to it. The retained stool becomes larger and drier, almost defying expulsion. It may sit there like a croquet ball. The child ignores the call of nature, or he doesn't want the pain of passing such a big stool, so he decides never to have another movement again. A little bit of softer stool may pass around this "ball valve" obstruction and stain the clothing, or the peristaltic waves of the colon will extrude a bit of the stool, which becomes pinched off by the anal sphincter.

Diagnosis is easy by inserting a lubricated finger into the anus. The big stool can be palpated just inside the anal sphincter. To prevent this Level II mechanical problem from becoming a Level IV psychiatric problem, the chunk may have to be dug out or enemata given until the rectum is empty. Professional help may be needed.

An effort must be made to prevent future impactions. Sometimes just stopping ingestion of dairy products is enough to control the problem.

About 10 percent of hyperactive children, again usually boys, leak a little stool into their underwear. They usually do not have a desiccated stool in the rectum. It is now believed that their distracted brain does not always get the message from the rectum, and the rectum acts independently. Parents are amazed at how easily the mess disappears within a few days of starting a nutritious diet plus vitamins and no milk. The rapid disappearance is a negative function of the chronicity of the condition; the longer the child has had the problem, the slower the recovery. At the first sign of stool leakage of the four- or five-year-old, who may be too busy to take the time to have a decent BM in the toilet, some reward system for clean underwear might preclude years of frustration.

Whether or not psychiatric help is needed to overcome

the distress, it is essential to nourish the cortex of the brain so that it can perceive what the nether department is doing and send back its messages: hold the sphincter tight until the socially acceptable toilet can be used. The brain also should be able to perceive what the psychiatrist (or supportive parents) is trying to do.

Gas is present in the intestinal tract of the newborn baby all the way from stomach to rectum in the first few hours after birth. It is normal, and most of it is believed to be air the baby has swallowed. Some babies can have a lot of gas and seem comfortable: yet others can have a very small amount and appear terribly distressed (*see* Colic, above).

Parents should try to notice the relationship between cramps, abdominal bloat (tense, protuberant abdomen that makes a high note when thumped with a finger), and newly introduced foods. Daily colic and gas suggest a milk allergy (cow's milk in the mother's diet), swallowed air, or additives in the vitamins. Intermittent distress would suggest a fermentation or allergy to a food ingested in the preceding six to twenty-four hours (it takes about twenty to forty hours for a meal to pass from mouth to anus).

I am amazed how many parents continue to insist on a daily quota of a pint to a quart of milk for their children despite the easily remembered fact of milk intolerance in infancy. A child may have outgrown the severe colic, but the chronic gas, bloat, indigestion (the "nervous stomach" or "irritable bowel syndrome") continues until all the milk intake is discontinued.

If the gas passed is especially putrid, some protein fermentation by intestinal bacteria is usually to blame, and the elimination of meats would be appropriate. Some find that taking lactobacillus capsules or yogurt or cultured milk (remember the milk allergy) might help. Some have found that pancreatic enzymes with meals will aid the body in splitting the proteins into absorbable amino acids before the bacteria ferment them.   The B vitamins will make the body "work better" and help the intestines manufacture the proper enzymes to do the splitting of the protein more naturally.   Some people find that B complex vitamins made from yeast are very gas-forming, so they change to rice polishings as the source of the B complex.

Gas from beans may be reduced by refrying them or by cooking them with sodium bicarbonate.   If one has gas and craves and eats some particular food daily, that food is probably the cause of the gas.

Ileitis or regional enteritis is a bowel inflammation that leads to scarring and narrowing of the passageway and even obstruction and perforation.   The disease starts quietly, with attacks of discomfort, nausea, gas, and cramps; it is usually thought to be the flu.   But it doesn't go away.   The patient feels tired, must rest frequently, avoids school; he may run little or no fever and hence he is called a malingerer.   A sedimentation rate and blood count usually reveal the true nature of this potentially serious disease.   The sed rate is up, the patient is usually mildly anemic, and the x-ray may show areas of dilatation and narrowing of the lumen of the ileum (part of small intestine).   Patients appear pale and have sunken eyes. Ileitis is considered an autoimmune disease like glomerulonephritis, rheumatic fever, and ulcerative colitis.   The suggested treatment is long-term use of cortisone.

This treatment puts the patient into a Level IV situation from which he may never rise.   Cortisone is a last-ditch medicine and as far as possible should be used as a temporary, short-term emergency aid.   If all signs indicate that the patient has ileitis, and if cortisone is the drug of choice and the patient is not completely bedfast, an attempt should be made to revive the exhausted adrenal glands.   The assumption is that if cortisone is helpful in controlling the problem, then the patient is not producing enough adrenal gland hormone because of diet, injury, disease, or some physical or psychic stress. Since we know how to nourish the adrenals, that method should be attempted first, before replacement cortisone is prescribed. Cortisone *is* effective here, but it is also a trap. The patient feels better in a few days; cheek color improves, the sedimentation rate falls, the hemoglobin level rises, and activity returns to normal. But any attempt to reduce the cortisone reveals the disturbing fact that the patient cannot maintain the improvement without the cortisone. He is hooked.

He may even be worse than before if the cortisone is terminated, because of the way cortisone works. Cortisol, the cortisone precursor circulating in the bloodstream, informs the pituitary gland as to its concentration. If the concentration of cortisol falls, the pituitary sends out more adrenal corticotrophic hormone (ACTH) to stimulate the adrenals to make more. If the cortisol concentration rises, the pituitary cuts down on its stimulating hormone. If, then, cortisone is supplied by mouth or injection, the pituitary assumes that it is time to reduce the ACTH. The adrenals, already exhausted, reduce their cortisone production and are unable to produce enough to control allergies, autoimmune diseases, or just the normal metabolism of all the cells of the body. The patient becomes cortisone-dependent. Although the therapy is slow and doesn't always work as we would like, it is worthwhile to supply supportive nutrients to the adrenals to help them resume their proper supportive functions, that is, making their essential hormones. The Prevention Diet is mandatory.

In ileitis, big doses of vitamin A, pantothenic acid, vitamin C, and all the B complex vitamins, especially B_6, should be supplied for months. The sedimentation rate, the blood count, and possibly a follow-up x-ray might be used to monitor the progress of recovery. If irreversible scar tissue has formed in the intestines, surgery may be necessary. If cortisone has been used because the situation was bad enough to require it, the above supportive measures may allow the cortisone to be reduced gradually to a dose that might not cause growth retardation or the characteristic "moon face" or the tendency to diabetes. Even if cortisone is being taken, it is possible with the adjunctive therapy to cut the patient's dependency on it. Zinc may help the intestines heal.

It is assumed that the disease would not have become manifest if the patient had not been suffering from stress or a poor diet for the years prior to the onset of symptoms.

Intestinal flu strikes most of us once a year, but adequate nutrition can reduce the frequency, severity, and duration of the illness. (Typically, it lasts seven days in children and twenty-four to forty-eight hours in adults).

In a child, the flu attack usually begins suddenly with vomiting that lasts about twenty-four hours, usually not long enough to cause serious dehydration. Then the other end explodes and cramps and diarrhea begin, lasting seven days. If possible, when flu is identified in the family, the remaining healthy members should saturate themselves with vitamin C and the B complex. It might help protect them or reduce the severity if they get it. Once flu begins, small sips of fluid containing salt, sodium bicarbonate, honey, and vitamin C should help replace the fluid losses, if the victim can hold the fluid down. No solids. About a quart of fluid should be swallowed every eight to ten hours. If the child is urinating 1 to 2 ounces three to four times a day, and if he can hold his head up, he probably will recover without further complications. But continued vomiting and diarrhea and fever make hospitalization worth considering.

Intravenous injections of vitamin C (1000 mg) and B_6 (100 mg) will sometimes stop the problem in its tracks. Some patients will sit up and ask for food even before the infusion is completed.

In any event, the disease is a stress and should be so treated. The assumption can be made that the patient would not have succumbed in the first place if he had been in adequate nutritional balance. Therefore, the weakness leading to the disease *and* the disease itself mean that the victim needs double the usual stress supports to bail him out. He may have to continue higher than usual nutritional supports for months to make sure he maintains himself at Level III.

Mesenteric adenitis is an inflammation of the lymph glands in the abdomen that usually strikes between ages two and six. It is difficult to recognize since the glands cannot be palpated. The illness can be mistaken for appendicitis because of an elevated white blood count and local tenderness; on operating, the surgeon finds enlarged lymph glands in the supportive membranes of the bowel—and a normal appendix. Somehow an infection has gotten into these nodes, and although the infection usually subsides by itself, it does suggest that the usual measures for infection should be used (vitamin C, especially). An antibiotic might be prescribed by the doctor, but does not preclude the stress, so it would be especially important to start the Stress Formula as soon as possible after the anesthesia has worn off.

Sometimes children with mild mesenteric adenitis are thought to be malingerers or to have a food allergy. Any constant pain in the abdomen, especially if it is accompanied by local tenderness or tight muscles (guarding the inflammation inside), should be evaluated by the doctor, who will probably check for an elevation of the white cell count (and possibly also of the sedimentation rate—*see* Ileitis, above).

Obesity in many cases is traceable to genetic factors. If both parents are obese, four out of five of their offspring will have to fight obesity all their lives. One out of five of the children of thin parents will note the same difficulty. Habit, taste, and social and emotional factors all contribute to the difficulty.

Studies show that heavy people tend to have higher insulin levels after carbohydrate ingestion; the insulin helps put glucose into storage as fat, where it is less available for energy needs. When fat people try to starve themselves into thinness, they lose weight, but most (65 percent) of the weight loss comes from the protein in the muscles, which only weakens them further. The trick, then, is to identify those who are more likely to manufacture too much insulin in response to carbohydrate ingestion and not let them even smell a quick calorie.

Stress is another factor in obesity. When stress drives the blood sugar down, the victim may respond to the resulting hunger sensation by eating something sweet; if his pancreas in turn responds with insulin, his blood sugar will fall again, not from stress this time, but from the responsive functioning of his pancreas. Emotional factors have thus initiated a genetic-biochemical chain of events. It also must be remembered that when the blood sugar falls, hunger is felt at a time when the neocortical control cells are poorly nourished. The victim figures "What the hell?" and has another attack of the munchies. Psychotherapy may be helpful for the problem that got it all started, but if no attention is paid to the insulin–blood-sugar cycles, little progress can be made.

Some people develop hypoglycemia (low blood sugar) as a result of food allergies, notably to corn, potatoes, and milk. When they eat these foods their blood sugar falls, adrenalin flow is stimulated, and they feel anxious; this is often seen in hyperactive children. Experience has taught these people to eat these same foods in order to get immediate, albeit temporary, relief. This is the basis of the allergic-addictive syndrome. The food one loves is the food one should avoid. Try to explain *that* to a surly, negative teenager. This can sometimes be demonstrated dramatically by placing a few drops of the extract of the craved food under the tongue. Within ten to twenty minutes the sensitive patient will have a pulse rate increase and become mute, aggressive, restless, paranoid, or "out of sorts." A smaller amount of the extract given now will abort the attack, presumably by raising the blood sugar to normal levels again.

If the patient has not yet escaped from the doctor's office, his blood sugar can be monitored; fluctuations of up to 400 mg and down to 40 mg in the space of an hour or so have been recorded. Some authorities now feel that perhaps 50 percent of diabetics and epileptics are misdiagnosed because *this* mechanism is the real basis for their symptoms. One can see the relationship of this phenomenon not only with weight problems but also with crime, hyperactivity, amnesia, migraine, schizophrenia, child-battering, rape, and, of course, alcoholism.

We doctors have not been asking the proper questions. We were taught that obesity is a matter of eating more calories than the body burns up; the excess is merely stored. However, the specific foods that are being consumed may be as important as their calorie concentration. The somatopsychic aspects are as important as the psychosomatic aspects.

A Level I child has some built-in mechanism that allows him to eat just the proper amount for growth and energy and to burn up what he does eat. He is neither thin nor fat. He has neither too much activity nor too little for his age or occupation. His parents are of normal weight for their height.

A Level II child might add a few pounds or become chubby if he is forced to remain indoors and inactive during a cold winter. Some feedback mechanism is not working efficiently enough to tell him not to eat so much when his energy requirements are less. An effort should be made to get him off a three-meal-a-day schedule in favor of five or six small protein-vegetable-nut-salad feedings a day. If his relatives are a little heavy, they should all be doing this anyway or they may all slip into Level III.

In a Level III obesity tendency, the family trait is fairly obvious in at least half the child's relatives and there is social pressure to "Finish your plate," "If you are good you may have some dessert." These children frequently have grandparents who believe "Sugar is love" or "One little cookie won't hurt"; it's plain to see from these grownups' waistlines that they are hooked on sugar. The danger here is that their grandchildren may have inherited the same tendency to hyperinsulinism. Many of these children soon acquire the philosophy that they cannot eat anything if it is not sweet.

Parents should make every attempt to nurse the baby who has these family traits and not begin solids until the child is close to nine to eleven months old. The solids that are introduced should be homemade if possible (mashed peas, beans, spinach, whole-grain cereals, eggs, lamb—one new thing a month). No puddings or desserts, and fruits and starchy vegetables only sparingly. Wheat germ, brewer's yeast, and desiccated liver powder should be laced into the foods and fed with a smile. The child is supposed to believe that sweet foods are rare and eaten only with protein foods. Only 2 percent milk in the cup. Water is the best fluid; serve fruit juices only occasionally. Continue indefinitely with the Prevention Diet.

A child who rolls into Level IV despite all of the above has a special metabolic problem which could be the result of genetic and intrauterine factors. Most plump infants slim down after eighteen months, and their weight (in pounds) is usually less than their height (in inches). For example, a satisfactory two-year-old girl might be 33 or 34 inches tall and weigh approximately 25 to 30 pounds. If the pounds equal or exceed the inches, obesity is getting to be a problem. Rule: If a child looks fat, he or she *is* fat. This Level IV child may also have a lifestyle of lethargy, sleeping in, indolence, thumb sucking, play avoidance, watching television for hours without moving. It is impossible to decide whether this sluggishness is the cause of the fat accumulation or the result of high carbohydrate ingestion and overproduction of insulin which shunts the energy into storage. It is amazing how these children know at such a tender age which foods are packed with calories. They love white bread, pasta, mashed potatoes, gravy, sugary cereals, sweets, candy, fruit, ice cream; usually they hate vegetables, salads, fish, and liver. They are frequently constipated because they cannot seem to eat any roughage. The weight of a full colon could promote the lethargy. The parents fall into the trap of letting them eat these things, for if they try to starve them into eating more nourishing foods, the children will eat nothing and as a result are likely to get sick, more tired, or downright mean. The path of least resistance is to serve them their favorites. Children like this are usually found in families whose life centers around food, so the child is trapped by these forces as well as by his own biochemistry.

Something *has* to be done for these children early to save them from the taunts of their peers as well as from the bad image they have of themselves. In adolescence they try to fast but only get sick and hate themselves because they haven't the self-discipline to lose weight. When they try any reducing program, they get the shakes because their blood sugar drops from all that insulin, and when the blood sugar is down, the self-control section of the neocortex is no longer operative. At this point, the eating center in the animal limbic system pushes them into the candy store.

Doctors can help, but a supportive group such as Weight Watchers works better. The whole family should be on a control program. With children, it seems to be easier to keep them from gaining so much as they grow rather than trying to make them lose (which could even be dangerous during the growing years). Many of these fat children will gain six to twelve pounds a year; if we can keep it under six pounds a year, we figure we have a chance.

Something more than the Prevention Diet usually is needed. It appears that the B complex vitamins help to metabolize the carbohydrates entering the body and serve to get some of it out of storage. B vitamins, especially niacinamide, can raise the low blood sugar levels that make these people tired and hungry. They need the stress amounts (200 mg of each of the Bs) and they need an exercise program. No promises should be made or given, just that they will feel better, have more energy, and look better. Don't set a goal about the child losing so much weight in so much time; instead, emphasize the concept of growing into the weight. Protein powder mixed with fruit or vegetable juice may be a valuable aid, but never follow an exclusively protein diet; this is too dangerous, even for adults.

Some effort must be made to discover and eliminate the child's most favorite food; that food could be a factor in causing the low-blood-sugar attacks and cheating that almost always accompany weight-loss programs. Turning off the television set will help, too.

Most parents of fat children hope that the obesity is due to low thyroid function, but it almost never is. Such children are frequently warm, flushed, and of average or above-average height. But Dr. Broda Barnes points out that the blood levels of thyroid hormone may not be an accurate way to determine thyroid function. He suggests taking the basal temperature before arising in the morning. Consistent oral or axillary temperature of less than 97.6 degrees might suggest a trial of thyroid extract for a month or so, if the family has been as conscientious as possible in following all the dietary rules we have recommended.

Pinworms are one of the most common causes of abdominal pain in children. These white quarter-inch-long pests live in the large bowel. The female migrates out of the rectum at night to lay her eggs about the anus. The resultant itch makes the child scratch. He picks up the microscopic eggs under his nails and then reinfects himself or passes them on to his friends by direct or indirect contact (toys or food). Eighty percent of children have pinworms at some time; repeated attacks are common. There is no immunity, although some feel that a well-nourished body and a healthy intestinal tract will not allow worms to survive.

The giveaway in the diagnosis is to observe the adult females crawling out of the child's anus about an hour after he has gone to sleep. Like a snipe hunter, the parent sneaks in with a flashlight, spreads the buttocks apart, and tries to get a look.

Doctors sometimes insist on more positive laboratory evidence before they prescribe vermifuge. The parent is asked to pat the sticky side of transparent tape against the anal opening first thing in the morning to pick up eggs laid during the night. The tape is folded together and mailed in to be examined under a microscope.

Sometimes it is best to treat the whole family and the child's friends simultaneously. But, for some reason, doctors refuse to believe how common the condition is and will not treat if it is merely suspected.

If the symptoms of anal itch, stomachache, teeth grinding, and restlessness during sleep do not permit your doctor to prescribe the very effective vermifuge for your family, you could try gentian violet tablets, garlic tablets, herb teas, snug underwear for sleep, short, scrupulously clean fingernails, and soap and water cleansing of the anal area every morning for two weeks. The worms only live six weeks in the body, and if one can break the reinfection cycle, they will die out.

Pyloric stenosis is the not uncommon condition of hypertrophy of the muscles at the exit of the stomach with resulting narrowing of the lumen and symptoms of obstruction. It is usually found in a firstborn male delivered in the spring

months. The vomiting begins early, before he is a month old.
It becomes projectile in just a few days and is not bile-stained.
Once it is fully developed it usually demands surgery because
dehydration can follow rapidly.

The surgery is designed to be as nontraumatic as possible. Under light or local anesthesia, the abdomen is entered,
the swollen muscle identified and cut down to the mucosal
lining. As soon as the baby can suck and swallow, he is allowed to eat and usually recovers beautifully, gaining weight
rapidly.

In this illness, a newborn who seems to be operating at
Level I can drop to Level IV or V in just a few days. He could
return to Level II in just a few days, but there is sound evidence to indicate that early surgery (stress) leads to a higher
incidence of allergy (hay fever and asthma) as the child
grows. It suggests that the adrenal glands became exhausted
from the vomiting and the subsequent surgery. Study also
suggests that it would be prudent to shore up the adrenals
with the Stress Formula to preclude the development of allergies.

It should be easy to get 100 to 200 mg of vitamin C down
this ravenously hungry baby. The vitamin B complex, with
20 to 50 mg of each of the Bs a day, is about right; B_6 and
pantothenic acid are the most important ones. After a month,
these doses could be cut in half, assuming the parents have the
child back to at least Level II. If the mother of a child with
pyloric stenosis is nursing this child, she should express her
breasts, bring the milk to the hospital and insist on its being
given to the child so that cow's milk will not be used.

Thyroid function has been studied for years. Low thyroid function usually manifests itself in fatigue, pallor, puffiness, coldness, slow heart rate, constipation, and dry skin because the thyroid hormone is involved in the metabolism of
every cell in the body. It helps get nutrients into the cells and

then catalyzes the cells' energy-producing system, a *sine qua non* of life.

One might suspect an inadequately functioning thyroid gland in a child because the child fails to grow satisfactorily. But genetic factors, anemia, lead poisoning, insufficient zinc intake, and low-protein diet all can play a role. If chronic infections, nutritional factors, and anomalies can be ruled out or corrected, then a thyroid workup might be helpful for short, cold, pale, waxy-skinned children who are also constipated.

A fairly accurate home thyroid function test is made by taking the oral or armpit temperature for five minutes before the child stirs out of bed. If the temperature is consistently 97.6° and below, it suggests the thyroid gland is not putting out a sufficient amount of its hormone; 97.8° to 98.2° is considered normal. Higher values suggest an oversecretion.

The low thyroid function may be due to hypoglycemia, poor intake of vitamins A, B, and C and iodine and some minerals, lack of stimulation from the pituitary, or an infection of the gland itself. It is important that proper nutrition and supplements be given for a month or so before deciding to try the desiccated thyroid as a replacement therapy.

If the morning temperature does not rise with the proper nutrition in a few weeks and a hair test does not reveal significant low levels of iron, copper, zinc, chromium or molybdenum, then a month of 1 or 2 grains of desiccated thyroid daily would be worth a try. (This is made from the thyroid glands of animals. Desiccated thyroid has been used for almost every ill known to man, occasionally with dramatic results).

If insomnia and diarrhea occur, the dosage should be cut back.

Ulcers are rare in children, but, when found, are almost exclusively localized in the duodenum, the 3 to 5 inches of small bowel just beyond the stomach. The anatomic relationship suggests the cause of the trouble: acid from the stomach squirts into the alkaline duodenum and burns a hole in the lining. This causes pain in the upper central area of the abdomen (or maybe a little to the right of upper center). If it continues, bleeding, anemia, or perforation (exquisite pain requiring surgery) may occur.

Genetics play a part in the etiology of this disease. I knew a five-year-old boy with an ulcer who appeared rigid about his daily habits (just like his uncle). Every night when he got ready for bed, he would carefully hang his shirt over the back of the chair, fold his pants neatly on the seat of the chair, hang his socks on a rung of the chair, and retie his shoes, which he placed side by side under the chair. Parents like neatness, but this was compulsive behavior. His parents had never even suggested to him how to dress or undress; his mother admitted that she left her clothes carelessly strewn about the bedroom. Her brother, however, had always been overly neat and did develop an ulcer.

The teaching in medical school was that stress was the primary initiating event that caused the hyperacidity, and that the twinges in the duodenum were the tears of the subconscious. The patients, usually men, were unable to vent their hostility, so it "backed up," becoming a somatic symptom. Genetics determined which organ would be the target.

The announced treatment seemed logical: antacid preparations and small, bland feedings of milk, cheese, eggs, and custards would neutralize the acid condition. Also, something had to be done to get the patient to express hostility without guilt. The treatment was generally effective because the pain subsided when the proper amount of acid was neutralized. But the recurrence rate was too high, so surgery—removing the acid-secreting area of the stomach, or cutting the nerves that stimulated the acid cells—was devised.

Then some field studies were done that caused thoughtful doctors to question the basic philosophy of this medical management. The studies seemed to indicate that ulcers did not develop in severe stress conditions if the diet contained only foods with a high buffering capability, that is, raw vegetables. Dr. T. L. Cleave, in his well-documented book, *The Saccharine Disease*, points out that soldiers under the stress of siege did not develop ulcers when they ate raw beets, potatoes, cabbage, and other foods they scrounged from the countryside. He figures that if the acid in the stomach were buffered properly with unprocessed food, that food would be chemically neutral when it was pushed into the duodenum; the duodenum would not be irritated and would be able to continue its alkaline digestion.

Although Cleave's treatment was contrary to orthodox medical management, his patients all healed promptly and recurrences were rare, despite the lack of treatment for the psychological stress. The patients were given no sugar or processed food; they ate raw or slightly cooked vegetables, cereals, seeds, nuts, and animal proteins.

Cleave theorized that the stomach secretes acid in response to substances in the stomach. If the material is sugar, white bread, or overcooked food, the acid secreted is not buffered sufficiently and this acidic material overwhelms the alkali in the duodenum. Many patients are reluctant to put roughage into their stomachs, assuming that these "harsh" materials will punch a hole in the thin ulcer base. However, it is only the acid that penetrates the mucosa; coarse food is well tolerated. If no food is presented to the stomach, no acid is produced. The small bits of bland food usually recommended to be swallowed frequently only serve to continue the acid production, and because the acid is not buffered properly, it continues to burn. This treatment usually prolongs the problem— if it didn't actually cause it in the first place.

Thus a child would be at risk for ulcers if he (1) is an overachiever or is overly neat, (2) comes from a family where ulcers are not uncommon, and (3) has a high-up stomachache which is relieved by food or antacids.   An x-ray may only show an "irritable duodenum," but attention must be directed to the diet.   Also, it is not uncommon to find that this irritability comes from an allergy to milk (especially to milk in a processed state); the prescribed milk may be the cause of the distress it is supposed to cure.

Call your doctor, obviously, but to keep your child (and you) from slipping down through the health levels, try the Prevention Diet, and just in case there is some stress in the environment, use the Stress Formula.   In a few days the symptoms should be gone or going.   If not, then something other than a sensitive duodenum is causing the pain.

Vomiting is the return of stomach contents which the victim thought were safely on their way to becoming nourishment.   Even a Level I person might throw up, but probably not more than once every two years.   Usually vomiting is the first sign of intestinal flu.   The victim slows down his activity, turns pale, has greenish eyelids, stares into space, opens his mouth, from which saliva runs out, and then lets fly.   The smart parent should be able to see it coming and get the child outside or bent over the toilet.

1. You could assume it is intestinal flu, if (1) the nausea and vomiting continue for twenty-four hours, (2) the child feels well enough to sit up and move around, and (3) the abdomen is soft and nontender to palpation (it should feel like kneading dough).

If the vomiting is projectile, intestinal obstruction must be considered.   If the vomiting is only in the early morning and is associated with headache, some pressure on the brain might have to be looked for.   Vomiting is common at the onset of any febrile disease. Just at a time when a body needs extra nourishment because of the stress of the disease, it is unable to hold food down. If you cannot get your doctor to give an intramuscular or intravenous injection of vitamin C, try to get sips of the following vitamin C drink down between the waves of nausea: dissolve one teaspoon (2½ grams) vitamin C powder in 3 ounces (about 100 cc.) of water. Two teaspoons of this solution will provide 250 mg of vitamin C. This amount every hour or so should help the patient fight off the virus. (It can be added to some other juice to make it more palatable.)

In the last twenty years, since antinausea medicines have been incorporated into suppositories, fewer children have required hospitalization and intravenous fluids. When the medicated cylinder dissolves in the rectum, the medicine thus released is absorbed and goes to the vomiting center of the brain. Drowsiness is a side effect, but parents should not allow this nausea-free time to pass; an ounce of water, tea, apple juice—some fluid with some minerals in it—should get into the stomach, the intestines, and the blood stream at twenty-minute intervals to preclude the dreaded dehydration. Usually a body can tolerate twenty-four hours of little or no fluid intake, but if urination is less than two times a day, listlessness is constant, the skin is dry and inelastic, and the eyes appear sunken, intravenous fluids in a hospital are mandatory. □

Most poisonings occur between 4:00 and 6:00 P.M. The child is crying out for something to eat because of a low blood sugar level. Give him half of his supper at 3:00 P.M. You may save his life.

The 9 Major Network

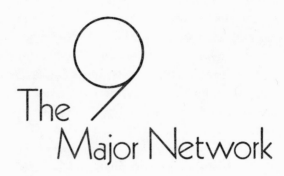

Nervous disorders may be the most alarming problems parents have to cope with in bringing up their children, possibly because they seem so mysterious in origin and because delicacy and patience are required in treating them.

I believe that these problems are not so insoluble as we once thought. Understanding the roles played by the limbic system (the animal brain) and the neocortex (the thinking brain) gives us some insights into human behavior. By keeping the neocortex well nourished we can keep the behavioral balance on the side of rational response to incoming stimuli. All this gives hope for the treatment of nervous disorders. (*See also* p. 130.)

The neocortex, the topmost layer of the cerebral hemispheres, is the repository of perception, cognitive function, conscience, and much memory. All these human and humane functions separate us from the animals around us and, we hope, are strong enough to keep a damper on the animal within us.

The animal brain, the limbic system, or the emotional brain is a combination of nuclei and nerve fibers situated between the cortex and the spinal cord and serves to modify or augment sensory stimuli from the outside world. If the neocortex fails to function properly, the animal brain takes over. And if the animal brain allows too many external stimuli to get through its elaborate filtering device, the neocortex may be overwhelmed by these stimuli and perceive that a crisis is imminent.

A working hypothesis is suggested: Dr. Jekyll behavior must be a function of the neocortex and Mr. Hyde (selfish, mean response) a result of the limbic, animal system taking over. How can we keep the neocortex constantly functioning so our children will perform in a socially acceptable way? How do we lock them into niceness? We are told by the behavior modification experts to reward good behavior and disregard the unacceptable. But if the neocortex is working only part time, it is frequently difficult to catch the fleeting positive moments.

Nervous system activity is the result of nerve cell depolarization; an impulse of electrical activity travels along the nerve fiber. When it reaches the end of the nerve fiber a chemical is released which is able to stimulate the next nerve fiber in the sequence. Enzymes supplied with the proper amounts of oxygen, glucose, amino acids and ketones produce the chemical transmitters and the energy to do this work.

There is no energy stored in the brain, so these busy cells must derive all the energy required from the blood stream flowing through the brain capillaries at that particular moment. Muscles and the liver use the energy stored as glycogen; the brain does not have this capacity. This is the reason that one fourth of the blood pumped out of the heart goes directly to the brain. The brain is a very busy organ. And children have two to three times the energy needs of adults.

Therefore, if the child is anemic or does not eat properly, the brain will be unable to function optimally. If the body is under stress, the blood glucose will fall. If the person consumes sugar, he may produce too much insulin, and the blood sugar will fall, depriving the brain of its energy source.

Enzymes require vitamin C and the B complex vitamins and some minerals plus a *constant* energy supply for the production of the brain chemicals to permit nerve functions. The neocortex is the part most vulnerable to these deprivations. When it goes, the next layer to take over is the limbic system— the devil in all of us. Depending on genetic influences, learned patterns of response, age, previous insults, and the environment, a particular person will react in his own particular way.

Some get tired; some develop headaches, migraines, epilepsy, asthma, stomach-aches, incontinence, dizziness, tics, twitches, hives, arthritis, depression, and a host of psychosomatic disorders that can be explained by the failure of the neocortex to run smoothly.

And as the neocortex turns off, so the nice human, social good rules are "forgotten." The circuits for the memory of these attributes are not energized sufficiently. A Mr. Hyde is the result.

Parents should be willing to take stock of themselves and their family life. The aggressive, anxiety-ridden, or delinquent child is trying to tell us something about the deep sources of his unhappiness, and these rarely exist without contributing factors in his or her home life. Here is where a professional family counselor can be of great help. But remember, any change for the better in family interaction will be abetted by everyone's cooperating in a program of health-giving nutrition.

Aggression is characteristic of animals when marking out their territory and when hunting and killing prey. They become aggressive if interrupted during mating or when their young are attacked. We accept the aggressive behavior of animals as part of the natural order of things. In a human, unprovoked aggression is not socially acceptable and there are legal restraints against it.

All grades of aggression or hostile response to stimuli might be seen in one family or class, right down to Level V aggression. A Level I child or adult would become aggressive only if provoked unduly and if "turning the other cheek" did not dissuade the provocateur. At the other end of the ladder is the man who becomes furious if passed on the freeway. He takes out after the passer, forces him over, and beats him up. A Level IV or V child would be the four-year-old who, when asked "How are you?," responds by hitting the questioner. We expect a two-year-old to become frustrated when he cannot build a tower of blocks; when they fall over he turns to scribbling with a shrug, as if to say "Maybe next week I will be able to do it." But if he begins to scream and throw the blocks at his sister, as if she and not gravity were responsible for the collapse, he has lost control and is at Level IV for aggression, at least for that moment.

Age is obviously a factor in aggressive behavior: the three-week-old baby who is mad because he is hungry is acting his age. He has no neocortical ability to delay gratification. But if he is operating at Level I or II, he will be able to ignore his hunger pains if he can see or hear his mother preparing to feed him. He is comfortable and secure and trusting; he and his mother have a mutual understanding, and the love that she demonstrates gradually becomes incorporated into his brain so that as he grows he operates in a socially acceptable way because his mother has become his conscience, his superego. That becomes fixed in his neocortex and if that goes, so does his "internalized" mother.

It is obvious that if a child is to develop a good self-image, the cortex has to be operating efficiently at the same time that the child's loved ones are demonstrating acceptance and love, or the child won't be able to perceive these environmental reinforcers. A poorly functioning or malnourished cortex will be unable to utilize this conscience or social regulatory system; it simply is not "lit up," so the limbic system, the lower animal, takes over. There is no reasonableness in the limbic system. It demands immediate gratification; everything has to go its way. No social concerns are found there.

Maturity in social response is based upon the development of the control department of the cortex. As the nerves of the brain mature, so does the child's ability to become a social human being with impulse control. Pediatricians are trained to observe this social awareness together with the child's physical and intellectual growth.

We expect the fifteen-month-old to have temper tantrums, but if a two-year-old continues to have these falling-on-the-floor responses to a simple "no," then he is called immature. His superego development has been sabotaged by an inconsistent or unaccepting environment or improper nutrition or "irritable focus" in the brain waves.

The ability to control aggressive, hostile outbursts is the hallmark of a mature human nervous system. This control requires a functioning neocortex and an accepting environment that reinforces and rewards socially acceptable behavior. If the neocortex never functions or functions capriciously, the environment (the parents) has difficulty rewarding and reinforcing that good, fleeting behavior.

Nutrition seems basic to the development of the mature human. If a child is a crabby, surly, touchy, noncompliant animal all the time, he may be suffering from worms, anemia, or odd brain waves. If his behavior is inconsistent and could be classified as "emotionally unstable" (Jekyll-and-Hyde), then it would be worth noting what foods were ingested in the one to twelve hours prior to a particular outburst.

It usually requires a stress—a question, a command, too

many stimuli, or a frustration—to trigger the action. In aggressive, noncompliant behavior, the stress is usually multiple: cutting teeth, plus eating sugar, plus ingestion of a known allergen (milk, wheat, citrus fruit, additives, corn, potatoes, nuts, and so on), plus some environmental stress (injury, surgery, perception of a threat), plus some genetic or congenital susceptibility (usually evidenced by ticklishness—see p. 225).

When these are dropped on a child all at once, he usually becomes hostile or falls on the floor or storms out or has a psychosomatic reaction (cramps, headache, asthma, hives, or "the flu").

If the Prevention Diet and Stress Formula are not allowing him to laugh and smile more than he cries and frowns, then a food-allergy elimination series should be attempted. (I assume that stress has been reduced.) Usually the food that is craved is the offender; if he loves milk and must have it every day, it is probably the milk that makes him feel out of sorts and unable to cope with stress.

The child or adult who responds best to the nutritional approach is the type who swings almost hourly from sweet compliance to wild combativeness with little or no environmental stimulus to explain the change. It almost always can be pinpointed to a food or carbohydrate overload within the preceding several hours.

The following gradations of unacceptable social behavior from Level II to V would be early warning signs suggesting chronic stress—either nutritional, physical, or psychic; it is a warning to the parents that something must be done so that aggression does not become a way of life.

The Level II child will fight only if provoked, if reprimanded will not repeat an unacceptable act, is usually cheerful when asked to do something, will help others voluntarily, is a good Boy Scout, brings lonely animals home. Level III is sometimes touchy, irritable, crabby, has occasional bad days, is noncompliant if not sure of success. Level IV is frequently surly, disappointed, defiant, sassy, needs to put others down, has temper outbursts, has few friends, hurts animals. Level V usually or always lashes out for no reason, hits, bites, scratches, throws or destroys toys, blames things on other people, has no give but lots of take, lies, cheats, and steals to win. When isolated in a room for punishment, he destroys the room; pulls a knife on mother when asked to do a chore; has no friends.

Any of the above can occur in any child or adult if the environment is hostile or unaccepting, if he or she has never developed a good self-image, if he or she has some chronic illness that demands close personal attention. The victim is so concerned about self that he has no time for nonself. He is just not comfortable; the world is too close and threatening. The space bubble that is big in Levels I and II is small and close-in at Levels IV and V.

Parents are delighted, of course, when the doctor discovers an ear infection to explain the surly behavior, but what if nothing is found? How far does a family push the doctor to search for some disease, infection, parasite, or chemical imbalance before saying, "Maybe you need a psychiatrist"?

The minimum workup before consulting a mental health professional should include:

Height and weight—if these deviate markedly from the norm for the age, some further testing of blood for thyroid function, blood sugar, anemia, lead and mercury levels is advised.

The following tests should be made: urine for kidney infection or anomaly; x-rays of bones for skeletal age; sweat test for cystic fibrosis; chest x-ray for heart anomalies; stool exam for malabsorption; glucose-tolerance test for blood-sugar peculiarities. The list could go on forever, but the history and examination would determine which tests would be prudent and appropriate.

Ear and tonsil infection, past or present, would mandate a trial of no dairy products for at least three to four weeks. A complete blood count, including the sedimentation rate, would help decide if a low-grade, subtle infection is present. If the sed rate is up and no obvious inflammation can be found, a trial of antibiotics might be considered.

Night wakefulness associated with surly behavior usually means pinworms. The double problem will be eliminated when the worms are. Continuing night terrors usually suggest an offending food or sugar ingestion prior to bedtime.

Allergy testing for foods and inhalants would be necessary if this type of child comes from an allergic family, has had severe colic, respiratory and intestinal infections in the past, or has nasal stuffiness or the tension-fatigue syndrome. His favorite food should be eliminated for three to four weeks as a test of the allergic-addictive phenomenon. The Ben Feingold diet should be tried for three weeks.

Dr. Feingold has found that much hyperactive behavior can be explained by allergies to aspirin, salicylate-containing foods, additives, colorings, and preservatives. (*See* Bibliography.) If it is only partially helpful, then the Basic Diet should be tried for three weeks. If staring or momentary loss of consciousness is suspected, a brain-wave test might be appropriate. If headaches are a prominent part of the symptomatology, a closer look at the nervous system is wise.

If tiredness and lethargy and lack of stamina are associated with the aggressiveness, the vitamin B complex, orally or by injection, should be tried.

If short stature, unmanageable hair, poor skin, acne, or white spots in the nails accompany the antisocial behavior, a trial of zinc (100 mg per day) for a month would give a clue as to that mineral's importance to the integrity of mental function. If sleep resistance, hyperactivity, restless legs, rocking, muscle and bone aches are related, then bone meal or dolomite should be tried—up to 1000 to 2000 mg of calcium per day.

We all probably need the sympathetic attention of a psychiatrist every once in a while anyway, but the psychiatrist cannot deal with the human limbic system. He or she must be able to talk to the cortex of the patient. (Psychiatrists should serve cheese and nuts in their waiting rooms.)

Many psychiatrists use nutrition as an adjunct to psychotherapy; they have found that psychiatric symptoms develop as a result of biochemical imbalances. Although nutrition may have improved the neurophysiology of the brain, the patient may be left with attitudes and defense mechanisms developed during the years of nutritional imbalance.

Anxiety is the feeling all humans have at times of stress and is usually the result of the flow of adrenalin. The heart pounds, the pupils dilate, nostrils flare, hair stands out on the back of the neck, muscles tense up, palms become sweaty—the whole body assumes an attitude of alertness and tension, ready for flight or fight.

This release of adrenalin from the adrenal glands into the bloodstream is stimulated by hormones from the pituitary and by nerve signals from the autonomic nervous system. The brain (cortex) perceives an environmental stress and sends a message to the pituitary gland, which does the rest. But the pituitary and adrenals have no way of knowing if the stress is worth getting all these juices flowing; these glands simply respond.

The cortex is the key, for it is *that* department that throws the switch, and if it is getting the wrong clues from the environment—a dysperception—it will be stimulating the pituitary and adrenals unduly. If a child or adult seems restless, tense, nervous, fearful, touchy, and if the environment does not appear to be so close or threatening as to justify all the response, the condition is called free-floating anxiety; it suggests a poorly operating filtering mechanism for incoming stimuli or a sensitive cortex. The sensitive cortex may not be able to handle the stimulus overload because it is not nourished properly.

All the cells in the brain require constant, optimum nourishment of glucose, amino acids, water, oxygen, vitamins, and minerals or they will not function. The brain has no storage capacity for energy as do the muscles and liver. The limbic system needs energy to filter properly, and the cortex needs it to process the information; the sheer volume of the incoming load may "panic" the cortex, causing it to overreact. Adrenalin flows.

The year-old baby who makes eye contact with the doctor is a good example. His immature nervous system cannot keep the doctor's gaze at a safe distance; he panics. But by age three, he has matured enough to look the doctor in the eye and even act friendly. But if he cannot make eye contact (because it is too scary), then he has anxiety, which may be due to a genetically poor filtering system, lack of other environmental supports, or some nutritional inadequacy.

Anxiety can result from psychogenic or nutritional factors because stress from these conditions will lower the blood sugar. A falling blood-sugar level will cause a release of adrenalin, and this release causes the bodily changes noted above. The nocturnal anxiety attack that makes the child scream out at two in the morning may be due to parental arguing, but it could also be the result of falling blood sugar from the dish of ice cream at bedtime. And this same falling blood sugar prevents the cortex from perceiving the "truth" of the environment.

A Level I child gets into new situations and finds that they are stimulating challenges. A Level V child is scared and sweaty even in the quiet of his secure living room surrounded by loving relatives. Reassurance does not help. He is a frightened rabbit. The world may be so frightening to him that he retreats to a safe inner world and becomes autistic, avoiding all human contact, relating only to objects, and developing rhythmical mannerisms to block out as many incoming stimuli as possible.

Anxiety Levels

Level I Joyfully plunges into new situations, school is fun, tries everything but is cautious if forewarned. Easy to toilet-train and not afraid to sit on the big toilet. Will try new foods but knows medicines are a no-no unless his parents say okay. Greets adults easily. Doesn't seem to be upset if parents quarrel occasionally.

Level II Not always reassured when parents say "It's all right." Tends to suck thumb or twist hair in new situations. A little teary on first day of kindergarten and first grade, but handles it well afterwards. Shy on introduction to adults but relaxes when he sees parents are comfortable.

Level III Somewhat ticklish but enjoys cuddling and holding. Didn't give up rocking or thumb-sucking until age five or six. Usually needs tranquilizer or sedative to get into new situation comfortably or go on a trip. Needs frequent reassurance: "How much farther?" "Will you come with me to the toilet?" "Brussels sprouts—yuk." "Tuck me in bed; someone is under my bed." Cuts and scrapes are serious: "Will I die?" Upset on days of appointment with doctor or dentist.

Level IV Won't come out of room if guests are present; trouble with eye contact and handshake. Will not enter in group fun at school, is at the edge of things even though his peer group is obviously enjoying the activity, a loner. Has to suck or rock to go to sleep until ten years old. Always dragging a blanket or doll around—has a tantrum if it's removed.

Eats only one vegetable. Very touchy, goosey, easily upset, a spook. Low threshold for pain or frustration and can't take a joke. Psychosomatic symptoms associated with stress, frustration, separations (headaches, stomachaches, asthma, hay fever, canker sores, bad dreams, depression and fatigue).

Level V Life is very serious, no sense of humor, paranoid, scared, misinterprets ("Are you talking about me?"). Notices own heartbeat: "Will I die?" "Are you going to die, Mother?" Many fears and phobias, special clothes and food necessary. Sits to one side in classroom, unable to respond when called upon. Won't enter big stores, won't ride bus, panics if left alone but cannot have people too close. Very sensitive to taste, smell, temperature changes. May be diagnosed as autistic.

The Level IV and V children usually are suffering from a neurobiochemical fault involving the screening mechanism in the brain. They may not be making enough norepinephrine in their limbic system. They may need Ritalin or another stimulant to initiate their production of that brain chemical. Their histories usually include prematurity, lack of oxygen, bilirubin excess after birth, or a traumatic delivery. They may have had encephalitis or meningitis as an infant or some toxic, surgical, or severe emotional stress.

Usually the supportive, basic nutritional program is not enough. Big and frequent doses of B complex vitamins—by injection,* if necessary—may have a calming effect, since they apparently increase the efficiency of the enzymes that manufacture the brain chemicals, especially norepinephrine. Niacinamide and pyridoxine (B_6) seem to be important here.

Many therapists have found the hair analysis for minerals helpful in deciding what to prescribe. Zinc often has been found to be low in the hair of these children; lead poison-

---

* 0.5 cc. of B complex intramuscularly every 2 to 5 days for 2 to 3 weeks.

ing can distort perceptions. Frightened, nervous, jumpy children are usually low in calcium and magnesium.

If the adrenal glands have been exhausted by the stress of chronic anxiety, allergies are often manifest because the cortisone-producing part of the adrenals has been overstimulated as well. In addition to the above, then, the allergy-control nutrients should be added—vitamin A, B₆, pantothenic acid, and vitamin C—to the Prevention Diet.

Exhaustion and depression easily can be superimposed on the anxiety and would, of course, be compounded by a carbohydrate diet which depletes the vitamins further; the resulting low blood sugar would allow the cortex to become even less able to receive the incoming stimuli.

Attention span is the most frequent reason given for a school referral to the doctor. If a child is distractible and jumps from one thing to another, he cannot learn well. Incoming information is not attended to long enough to be memorized, and it is not retained in his cortex long enough for optimal academic performance. Attention-span problems usually accompany hyperactivity either as a cause or an effect.

It may be the result of poor prenatal nutrition, premature birth, oxygen shortage at birth, difficult delivery, high bilirubin retention, brain infection, highly refined carbohydrate diet, insufficient intake of B complex vitamins, anemia, food allergy, lead poisoning, environmental stress, too many pupils in the classroom, tough teacher, low IQ, and so on.

If poor vision or hearing, anemia, and inappropriate placement in the classroom can be ruled out, a trial of the Prevention Diet and exclusion of additives and salicylates* must be tried. This approach takes about three weeks.

* Dr. Ben Feingold has found that a number of children are hyperactive because of an allergy to aspirin and salicylate-containing foods. (*See* Bibliography.)

A Level I child can do schoolwork despite a noisy classroom and looks up only when the teacher calls his name. A Level V child is distracted and cannot attend to a book or TV show even when alone in his secure, calm home. He appears inner-driven; he doesn't need an outside stimulus to distract him.

If the Prevention Diet is not sufficient to control this symptom, the B complex vitamins should be increased to 100 to 200 mg of each. If the attention span becomes shorter and the victim seems more restless and hyperactive, it suggests that there has been a histamine release and pantothenic acid, calcium, and magnesium are low and must be increased.

Many school children are given Ritalin, Cylert, or dextroamphetamine or other stimulants to control the attention span. If these substances are helpful, one assumes that the victim does not have enough norepinephrine in his limbic system. If a drug helps, fine; but that very fact indicates that the nutritional approach and extra vitamins also will help—and may even control the symptoms better and with fewer side effects than the drug. A trial of drugs, then, is worthwhile to discover this phenomenon. The B complex vitamins are essential to enable all the enzyme systems of the body to manufacture their chemicals in sufficient amounts. If not enough norepinephrine is produced the child (or adult) will have a short attention span and usually will be ticklish and hyperactive. Nutritious food and B vitamins (and sometimes zinc) help that enzyme in its work.

If the attention span varies from day to day or hour to hour, it suggests that the blood sugar is fluctuating because of sugar ingestion or consumption of food to which the victim is allergic. Physicians often forget to ask about diet, assuming it is not important here since lots of children eat "junk" and seem to do well in school. To investigate this, the mother and the teacher may have to work together, the teacher calling the mother with a negative report and the mother correlating this behavior with what the child ate for breakfast. It doesn't have to be sugar or white flour. Potatoes, corn, milk, MSG, or coloring in food or vitamins might be the stress that is reducing the blood sugar. Of course, this very stress uses up B vitamins at a faster rate and further decreases the enzyme that makes the norepinephrine in which this particular person is already deficient. A vicious cycle. Stress causes further stress.

Many teachers report that the class is attentive and calm until 11:30 A.M., or is doing well until after lunch. The child's brain has two to three times the energy needs of the adult brain, so even with a nutritious breakfast a child may need to eat a snack of nuts or cheese at about 10:30 A.M. The afternoon problem is usually attributed to the high amount of refined carbohydrates in the lunch.

Autism is a form of childhood schizophrenia. The cause is unknown, but may be multifactional. In general, the child so afflicted cannot relate to other humans. He seems to be responding to inner messages. He cannot maintain eye contact and has a variety of rhythmical mannerisms—rocking, humming, gesturing—that he repeats endlessly. It is felt that these activities serve to keep the world at a distance, as if the child is attempting to retreat from a confining or threatening environment.

Some cases are felt to be a form of brain damage. Some may be due to the child's psychological retreat from an emotionally painful environment (cold and punitive caretakers). Most investigators feel that a biochemical fault in the nervous system allows too many stimuli to get through the limbic screening section or to overload the sensitive neocortex where the ego perceives a threat. Retreat seems to be the safest response; autism is the only method a sensitive child can use to remove "himself" while still remaining physically in the uncomfortable environment.

A diagnosis of autism would be a Level V for shyness,

withdrawal, or retreat, so the same nutritional supports might be helpful. (This is not to say that a shy, frightened child will become autistic, merely that the same vitamins and minerals usually are used.)

A child I observed who came out of her autistic behavior was found to be low in zinc. She was short (less than 40 inches at age five years), had stringy hair and white spots in her nails. She was diagnosed as retarded, brain-damaged, or autistic mainly because she seemed to drift in and out of her own unique dream world. Within six months of starting the nutritious Prevention Diet, extra vitamins (especially B_3 and B_6), and zinc (90 mg per day), she had grown 3 inches (equal to a two-year increase in a normal child), her hair had become manageable, the white spots had disappeared, and she had begun to function in a normal, social, eye-contact way: "Hi, Mom, what do we do today?" It was learned that her father is a slow healer when cut, which frequently indicates inadequate zinc uptake. She was eating foods that easily gave her 15 mg of zinc a day, but her metabolism requires several times that amount to provide her enzymes.

A hair analysis was the key to finding this odd, rare deficiency. Zinc is not the universal answer, and this is only one case, but it illustrates the need for a more total analysis of such problem behavior.

Bedwetting (enuresis) has been defined as nocturnal emptying of the bladder in any girl over four years or any boy over five years of age. Diabetes, anomalies of the urinary tract, and infections should be ruled out before the child is labeled enuretic.

A Level I child is dry at night after eighteen months of age, despite stress, extra fluids, or deep sleep; he never wets the bed and has good control during the day. A Level V bedwetter wets himself during the day and may wet the bed two or three times during the night.

Although stress may cause the problem to occur occasionally in a Level II or III child, the every-night bedwetter is usually suffering from deep sleep caused by low blood sugar that is related to sugar ingestion or food allergy. The condition frequently is found in children who are allergic to milk or citrus foods—as if the bladder were sneezing. The problem should cease in these cases immediately after the offending foods are discontinued.

Some effort should be made to determine the child's bladder capacity; a capacity of at least 10 to 12 ounces is necessary if the child is to remain dry all night. Have the child wait as long as possible during the day, then measure the output. If the bladder capacity is under 5 or 6 ounces, perhaps this muscular balloon cannot stretch adequately. This may mean that there is not enough magnesium in the body. It is amazing how 500 mg of magnesium or a few dolomite tablets may stop the wetting almost overnight. Magnesium may loosen the bowels.

Many parents have used a bedwetting device with some success (a wired pad under the sheet allows an electrical current to close when the urine flows; a light goes on and a bell rings and the child is conditioned to awaken. He soon learns to awaken before this occurs). But he may sleep so soundly that the parents are up and standing at the bedside of this almost-unconscious child.

Hypnosis can work, too. A drug called imipramine is the usual prescription for this, but there are side effects, and it should be the last thing to try.

If a child wets only occasionally, the family should review the food, stress, and events of the previous day to see if some cause can be eliminated. In the typical situation, the somewhat hyperactive child is bribed with a dish of ice cream (20 percent sugar) to get him off to bed. The falling blood sugar at two o'clock in the morning prevents the cortex from getting the message from the bladder, so the latter acts independently. The irate parents tend to blame the child the next day, but at this time they are talking to the cortex, which never received any clue about the state of the bladder at 2 A.M. Blaming one end of the body for something that happened at the other end only serves to give the child a bad self-image. Telling a child he will become a criminal if he continues to wet the bed may encourage him to become a criminal; it never stops the wetting. Psychiatric problems are usually the result of the wetting, rarely are they the cause.

Biting is an aggressive act usually restricted to the one- to three-year-old who feels crowded. (One of our children bit a lady's behind when she moved back in a crowded elevator.) This seems to happen when there is poor cortical control of impulsive behavior combined with difficulty in verbalizing feelings.

A Level I child would only respond with biting if he were attacked when hungry or tired and if the attacker were not dissuaded with a smile.

A Level II child would bite from age ten months to twenty months during the time of tooth eruption, but only if stressed or threatened. He drops this physical aggression when he is able to counter aggression verbally. "I hate you" would be a verbal attack and more socially acceptable than biting. He is learning.

The Level III child continues to bite after age two years and for little or no provocation. It is difficult to use psychology on a child when one's arm is being eaten; quietly placing the child in the time-out room for fifteen minutes is the best thing to do at such a time. To deal with the problem, one should sit down and (1) make a list of everything the child ate for the past two to six hours, and (2) decide how stressful was the inciting stimulus. Usually low blood sugar or food allergy must be present for a stimulus to trigger the aggression.

The Prevention Diet and vitamin additives should be satisfactory to stop the problem.

In Level IV, the child feels punk most of the time and doesn't care whom he bites. He seems to have a chip on his shoulder. No external stimulus is needed to trigger the biting. If he has occasional good hours or days, a nutritional problem is more likely to be causative. Usually the Level IV child is very shy or very hyperactive or very allergic or very pale. His appearance and behavior suggest a course of action to include diet change, no milk, extra vitamins, calcium, magnesium, blood tests, and a search for infection.

If he has slipped to Level V despite nutritional intervention, he may be acting like a caged leopard, snarling and biting at anyone who comes near. Pouting, kicking, fighting, screaming is his response to "Good morning." We must control the natural impulse to fight back and realize that this is a sign of severe depression, bad self-image, lead poisoning, or unhealthy or unsupportive environment.

We try all the tricks here: fasting for three days, no milk, vitamin B injections, electroencephalogram, hair analysis, blood tests and sedimentation rate for infection, moving the child out of the home into foster care for a month or so. Psychiatric evaluation or drugs may be necessary. There is some evidence to indicate that antisocial behavior is reinforced by the attention it gets, even if negative (*see* Aggression, above).

Clumsiness is usually considered an innate genetic or congenital problem. It is a soft neurological sign that may suggest a subtle hurt to the nervous system. A clumsy two-year-old may grow up to be a skilled athlete. It could be the result of being pigeon-toed or knock-kneed or flat-footed, but these are usually temporary structural problems that may be gone by age six years.

Some hyperactive children are very adroit, but some may

bump into things and fall because they directly approach everything they see. A child with scissors gait would tend to be clumsy because his cerebral palsy from a birth injury has destroyed many of the nerve cells that allow for smooth, voluntary activity.

A Level I child rarely gets cut or hurt or stubs his toe or falls over things or breaks a bone. He would make a good tennis player, quarterback, or shortstop because he has good eye-hand coordination.

A Level II child is active and robust but misjudges occasionally and bangs his head, scrapes his elbows and knees, and has had one visit to the emergency room for stitches somewhere.

If he is in Level III he is a caution. He is accident-prone partly because he is hyperactive and needs to win. The same hurt to the nervous system that produced his overactivity may have destroyed a few cells in the coordination department. As he grows, he learns to avoid the activities in which he is unsuccessful—usually those requiring good eye-hand coordination. The child or adult on this level could profit from the Prevention Diet plus the vitamin supplements; while it is true that some of the important nerve cells have been destroyed, there are still plenty of living cells nearby that might be made to function better if they were optimally nourished. The B complex vitamins, especially B_6 (100 mg per day), would be worth trying for at least a month to see if they can help him zig and zag better. Testing his vision also seems sensible. Have the ears tested for fluid.

Levels IV and V would contain those children who have some nervous-system defect such as cerebral palsy, hemiplegia, multiple sclerosis, polio, muscular dystrophy, hip dislocation, and the like. We know that the body or brain can lose much tissue and remain functional. It makes sense to try to stimulate or nourish the remaining cells to function up to their full potential. Dead cells are dead cells and cannot be brought to life, but I have seen severely crippled, stiff, bedridden, brain-damaged children show some purposeful movement or sign of recognition on their usually blank faces the day after a B complex injection.

A nutritional program plus vitamins and minerals should facilitate the physiotherapy.

Crying is expected of a child when frightened or hurt. Most adults would like to cry at times, but we are afraid we will be called immature if we do.

We feel the Level I child would cry at appropriate times: broken arm, cut lip, death of a loved one, very sad movie, mother walking out of room (up to ten months old; after that age he figures she is coming back soon).

A Level II child may cry on the first day of school (age five to eight years), at the doctor's office when the doctor examines him (age twelve to twenty-four months), when hurt, or if his parents fight. He will accept reassurance, however.

If he slips into Level III he will appear frightened most of the time. He perceives the world as a scary place and needs to be reassured—usually of his mother's presence. He would cry if momentarily lost in a crowd or when the doctor walks into the examining room. He is afraid of new foods, new experiences.

This child senses anxiety; he is fearful because of the extra adrenalin floating about in his body. He perceives the world as close and threatening. If all goes well, he is comfortable, so he may develop rituals that leave nothing in question where food, clothes, and schedules are concerned. His sense of humor is blunted.

A Level IV child cries at every new thing that comes his way. He is telling us that his filtering system is not working, the world is too close. Before he is given a tranquilizer to make him comfortable, an effort should be made to evaluate his environment and to strengthen the filtering activity of his brain.

Calm rocking, holding and loving are called for, and such verbal reassurances as "You are okay. We love you. Don't feel that way. We will never leave you." If excessive crying is associated with ticklishness, the conclusion is that the limbic filter is not working, and the Prevention Diet, the Stress Formula, and calcium and magnesium must be given. If the child is already on these, perhaps some blood tests, or heavy-metal poison tests, should be made. Testing for food allergy might be appropriate in some cases.

In Level V the problem may have to be treated by psy-chiatric intervention, but the nutritional program is essential at the same time, since the therapist can only deal with the cortex of the brain. In general, people who have fits of crying "for no reason" are almost always suffering from hypoglycemia due to sugar ingestion or food allergies. A fast may help. If it is a food allergy, the crying victim states on the third or fourth day of vitamins and vegetable juice, "I haven't felt this good for years." It doesn't always work, however. A brain-wave test might give a clue when everything else has been tried (*see* Anxiety, above).

Delinquency is usually the term used to describe the be-havior of the adolescent in committing aggressive, antisocial acts—running away, defying authority (parental or social), vandalizing property or setting fires, refusing to attend school —in general, breaking as many rules as possible.

His problem may well be a mixture of bad nutrition, boring education, unsupportive parents, and feelings of worth-lessness. The child (usually a boy) feels "What's the point of trying?" since no one appreciates what he does. He sits in class with his jacket on, his arms folded over his chest, a surly smirk on his face. The teacher cannot stand his look and challenges him. He gestures obscenely and is expelled. He concludes he is a bad person, since bad people are expelled. He continues his delinquent behavior and may go into adult crime.

Anyone who has dealt with delinquents is aware of the almost universal statistics: 75 percent of criminals were hyperactive children; more than half have abnormal glucose tolerance tests; 50 to 70 percent of criminals have a severe reading problem; and 50 percent of crime is related to alcohol ingestion. The delinquent who is truant and stealing is more likely to become an adult criminal if his father was a criminal or an alcoholic, suggesting some genetic influence.

These statistics might be lowered if we made school more interesting and offered individualized instruction. Some type of useful work should be provided for these youths so they can feel like worthy members of society. Reducing—perhaps even banning—the use of sugar and white-flour products would be a great step forward. The young adolescent is the one most susceptible to these quick carbohydrates because of his or her rapid growth between the ages of ten and fifteen years. The seventh grade seems to be the time of worst reaction.

A Level I adolescent is able to strike a balance between the pressures of his peer group to experiment with drugs, pot, alcohol, and antisocial behavior and the mandates of the conscience he has received from the parents who love and trust him. He has a good self-image, he has fun and is rewarded for doing socially acceptable things, so he doesn't have to fight the establishment at every turn. He has self-confidence and is able to laugh at himself. When he occasionally gets depressed, he eats something good for him, takes a nap and awakens refreshed.

An adolescent in Level II might try skipping school, stealing, or taking drugs, but these experiments don't make him feel any better, so he gives them up. He does like some of the people who do these things, but guilt prevents full participation. When his parents say "Don't," he quits, happily, but pretends to his friends that he is always being "pushed around." He experiments with alcohol—maybe wine—and a cigarette or two; those nauseate him but he is excited by the idea that he is doing something taboo. He might talk big to his peers about his prowess with drugs and girls, but everyone knows he's not that experienced. He wants peer acceptance but is afraid of the initiation rites. He starts to become negative toward his parents; he finds fault with how the food is cooked or the house is run. He breaks curfew. A thirteen-year-old daughter will want to date but will be comfortable if her parents say "Not yet."

In Level III the adolescent needs his peers more than his parents. He is stubborn and noncompliant but he does get to school. He acts as if the world, school, and home are a boring drag. He would sleep until noon if he could. He smokes, but not at home. He won't eat breakfast with his parents because he knows they will criticize his hair, clothes, attitude. He goes to school mainly to see his friends. A girl might wear provocative clothing or at least enough makeup to make her mother wonder if she is a lady of the night. Somehow these youths survive these years, but only luck seems to keep them out of close calls with drugs, cars, booze, and the police.

If we can keep these young people on a reasonably nourishing diet so that they feel good most of the time, they may not slip into Level IV.

A Level IV adolescent really does not feel good. He will do anything to feel "better": smoke pot, get stoned, eat junk. He believes nothing adults say. He has moments when he "surfaces" and is gentle, compliant, socially responsive, but the slightest pressure to do his homework, or help around the house, or stay home at night is met with surly noncompliance: "You're always bugging me. Get off my back."

In his efforts to be mature and cool, he may make a mistake and drink too much, drive too fast, go too far sexually and have to come crawling home, terribly embarrassed. Survival may be a matter of luck. A friendly, sympathetic doctor, minister, uncle, or school counselor may be able to catch him as he ricochets through the teen years. A nourishing diet would be helpful to keep the circuits in his neocortex operative, but usually he can't be stopped from reaching for the sugar and junk food that keep him functioning at his lower animal level.

Parents have to be understanding and try to move him toward a happier lifestyle. A nourishing diet will help smooth the way—if one can get him to eat it. Nuts, cheese, raw vegetables, fruit, bits of chicken, hard-boiled eggs, and seeds left out at strategic times and places might just keep his blood sugar up at a level compatible with normal brain activity.

In Level V delinquency, the behavior becomes a police matter. The story for years has been one of bad self-image, periods of depression, head- and stomachaches, pallor, bad complexion, erratic school performance, insomnia, allergies. All this should have alerted the parents, if not the doctor or school psychologist, that the child was going downhill somatically and consequently psychically to this almost irretrievable level. The early warning signs were there; how could we have failed to respond?

Thanks to a few far-sighted judges and court social workers who realize the biochemical origins of antisocial behavior, we can pick up a few of these deviants and set them straight.* Giving them good nutrition in a sympathetic foster home, instead of naked carbohydrates in a juvenile detention home, may be the only thing needed to get some of them on the right track.

Some community colleges will take sixteen-year-olds and fit them with a scholastic program designed to achieve high-school certification. Psychiatric intervention and tranquilizers

* Mrs. Barbara Reed, probation officer in Cuyahoga Falls, Ohio, is a pioneer in the understanding of the relationship of crime to hypoglycemia.

or mood elevators may be required for some. In any case, we cannot abandon these potentially useful citizens.

Depression seems inconsistent with childhood. A depressed child suggests an unaccepting home or a poor self-image. An aggressive, surly child who lashes out physically may be a depressed child protecting his collapsing space bubble. He may feel anxiety because he cannot cope with a threatening environment. A temper tantrum in a fifteen-month-old could be a depressed child's angry response to his perception of a loss of love.

Some children—and adults—respond to falling blood sugar with anxiety, fear, and depression simultaneously. Some will note a feeling of impending doom when their adrenalin starts to flow; tearfulness and withdrawal without sufficient reason calls for a review of the previous six to twelve hours' diet.

Level I children have sunny dispositions. They are likely to handle frustration and disappointment with a shrug of the shoulders and an "Oh, well!"

A Level II child will cry, turn away, and go to another room to hide his feelings.

Very slight insults and putdowns cause the Level III child to throw furniture or kick a hole in the wall or bash the cat. He may pout for a day or carry a grudge or stay in his room for a few hours. He cannot handle this kind of stress coming at a time when his blood sugar is at an ebb. A command or question at this vulnerable time is perceived as an overwhelming threat. With children who have this potential for negative response, parents (and teachers) would be prudent to ask for compliance only after a nourishing meal.

If parents discover their child is susceptible to sullenness, negativism, and depression, they should never deviate from the Prevention Diet and B vitamin supplements. Low blood-sugar levels will leave the neocortex more responsive to environmental stresses and feelings of inadequacy. The limbic system needs B vitamins to produce the brain chemicals that allow a nonthreatening environment to be perceived as such.

A Level IV child will appear frightened, withdrawn, and anxious so much of the time that his parents can rarely draw him out of his shell. He will be passive, a mere spectator to most events. Anything outside of his secure home will be a threat. A hair analysis might reveal some mineral imbalance which could be corrected; lead or mercury poisoning might be uncovered. Some withdrawn children may be low in zinc.

If the child sinks to Level V, it may be difficult to distinguish him from the autistic child, and psychiatric intervention should be sought. Antidepressant drugs may allow him to feel that the world is not so awful.

Childhood suicide is reported more commonly now and represents a failure of parents, school, and the medical profession to recognize the early warning signs.

Dizziness in a child is usually due to the failure of the inner ear to inform the brain properly as to the victim's position in space. This requires an expert evaluation by an ear-nose-and-throat specialist. If the doctor can find no infection, an allergic swelling of the inner ear structure might be considered; in such a case, consuming no milk, wheat, eggs, corn, or additives for a time might be curative. Heavy-metal poisoning would be the next consideration. A serious tumor would have to be searched for with an electroencephalogram or brain scan.

Dizziness is a subjective symptom, and it is difficult to make the diagnosis in a small child just by looking at him walk or run. Is he clumsy? Does he run into things in the semi-darkness (possibly due to a lack of vitamin A)? Perhaps he is hyperactive and literally plunges into new situations? Is it lightheadedness caused by anemia or low blood sugar? Is it fatigue because his copper or iron stores are down? Answering such questions will show the way to a cure.

Drug abuse is the term applied to the use of drugs to an extent far beyond their usual medical indications. Most of us gradually over our life span find some food, drink, or substance that we seem to need, that we have to have. Alcohol is the most commonly abused "drug," and 5 to 10 percent of adults in our country are considered alcoholics; they need it daily and manipulate their routine so that some alcohol can be ingested at regular intervals. The caffeine in coffee can be considered a drug. Some of us are hooked on sugar, chocolate, licorice, salt, even laundry starch; indeed, a syndrome called *allergic-addictive* is used to describe these people who insist that they have to have their favorite food or drink daily.

By finding the particular substance that someone craves, we can diagnose that person's unique biochemistry. We do not have to do a five-hour glucose tolerance test on someone who craves sugar; we know he has reactive hypoglycemia and that to correct the condition he must be taken off this "drug." It is estimated that 90 percent of alcoholics have low blood sugar. The condition pushed them into drinking, and the damage done to their pancreas or liver perpetuates the craving. If a coffee lover tries to go without his caffeine, he may get a terrible headache he knows can be cured only by drinking some of the hot brown stuff. The rule seems to be that if someone craves something, that something is bad for him.

Part of the explanation for an addiction to food is that an allergy to something in the food makes the blood sugar go up for a while and afterward to plummet downward. This subsequent uncomfortable feeling encourages the victim to ingest the offending food again. He is rewarded by a return of energy and sense of relief; he has learned what to eat when he feels depressed or out of sorts.

In a recent California study of a thousand women, half of whom were schoolteachers and the other half housewives, 80 percent of the blue- or green-eyed ones craved chocolate, coffee, or cola drinks. About half complained of frequent headaches. The women had discovered by some trial-and-error method that the caffeine (or theobromine or xanthine in the chocolate) had an antiheadache effect; they felt better when they took these "drugs"—possibly because stimulants act to release sugar from the liver. About 10 percent admitted that they frequently would down a whole can of chocolate syrup on the day preceding a menstrual period (a stress time when the blood sugar is traditionally low). Increasing the protein-nibbling and doubling the Stress Formula prior to menses should help. B_6 is very important.

From such food addictions it is not a big step to real drug addiction. Young adolescents frequently experiment with alcohol, marijuana, LSD, sleeping pills, tranquilizers, or inhalants such as gasoline or glue. Peer pressure, bad self-image ("Bad people take drugs. I'm bad; therefore I'll take something"), boredom, and a very real symptom—feeling miserable —set them up for these experiments. About 2 to 3 percent go on to heroin, cocaine, or alcohol. When they experiment, they get a rush of pleasure—"Boy, I feel great!"—an attitude that literally pushes them into continuing.

A Level I adolescent might try pot or alcohol because his friends are using it. This does little for him because he is in peak mental and physical health, and he doesn't like the altered perceptions of the environment that are part of the experience.

In Level II a person might grow up to like a glass of wine or a cup of coffee occasionally; he might even smoke a joint now and then, but it makes him nervous not to have full control over his own body, so he becomes very selective as to time and place.

Level III children and adults become almost boring

about the certain things they have to have every day: big glasses of milk, ten cups of coffee, chocolate ice cream, and so on.

Some effort must be made to help the Level III child or adult feel comfortable in his daily life, so that food craving or drug ingestion is not important to him. The Stress Formula is helpful. A no-sugar regime may prevent the drop in blood sugar that makes the victim crave something. At the same time, it may aid the conscience or superego (the self-control part of the cortex) in exerting influence over the limbic system (the pleasure-seeking area).

The Level IV or V adolescent has developed such a bad self-image that he tries to go from one high to another. Each intervening low forces him to get another fix. Recent evidence suggests that the use of 10 to 20 grams per day of vitamin C plus some supportive counseling may be helpful in getting the trapped person off his "junk." These people are so far gone that they usually have to be confined to a holding area for therapy.

Dyslexia is the term applied to anyone who has reasonably normal intelligence but difficulty in reading. Many hyperactive children are so distractible that their short attention span prevents the acquisition of reading skills. Some children have difficulty learning to read and this frustration causes them to be hyperactive. Hyperactivity can thus be cause or effect.

There are many types of dyslexia. Some children cannot remember the sounds of letters. Some have letter reversal (*god* is *dog*). To some the words dance on the page, while others can read but will not remember (see *Overcoming Learning Disabilities* by Martin Baren, *et al.*). A child who has difficulty learning to read at the usual age of six or seven years is said to have development dyslexia. This child usually will learn in time if he is not completely discouraged. Superficially, however, there is no reliable way to differentiate him from the ones who have a specific deficit. The latter group is divided into those who have a sensory impairment, a problem in processing sensory information, or a motor-expressive fault. Special reading-disability diagnosticians are needed to differentiate the groups. Therapy is designed to make use of what skills the child has to get messages into the cortex and out again. Normal speech development (indeed, normal motor and social development) usually is required to get the child to the point of being able to read.

The cortex or cognitive areas of the brain are essential to reading. Before the child is called stupid, an all-out effort should be made to nourish the brain optimally and continuously with the Prevention Diet and the Stress Formula. This would be especially important if the child has allergies, anemia, lead poisoning, brain damage, repeated ear infections, visual problems, or was born of a stressful pregnancy or delivery. The sooner the matter is investigated the better. Speech and reading are functions of the higher cortex and develop sequentially after early bonding with the mother, sitting, crawling, standing, walking, and so on. Learning waits on maturation, and the brain and the body work together toward maturity. The brain suggests an activity to the body; the body responds and sends messages back to the brain, which "sets" that activity in its "things accomplished" department. On the basis of this, plus reinforcement from the environment, the next idea is attempted.

A Level I child might teach himself to read because he has auditory memory and verbal skills and his perception of letters is clear. He easily associates and remembers the sounds of the letters of the alphabet at age three or four.

A Level II child may get most of these associations at age five years but needs a teacher to help him integrate these skills in late kindergarten or first grade. Once he gets it he becomes an avid reader. Supportive parents and a good diet should help.

A Level III child might be somewhat hyperactive and it would take him until age seven before he could consistently remember the difference between 3 and E. He may use "saw" instead of "was" and transpose letters—for example, "liltte" for "little." A special reading teacher should be able to straighten him out before he is eight years old. If he has good and bad days, his diet should be investigated as well as his hearing (audiometric test) and his vision (optometric examination). Is he anemic? Is his hyperactivity shortening his attention span? (All these difficulties should have been corrected a long time ago.)

A Level IV dyslectic child will require a special reading therapist on a one-to-one basis. If he is hyperactive, as is usual, he should have a minimum of extraneous stimuli in his environment so that his attention span will be as long as possible. If his diet has been altered (no sugar, no additives) and if he has a protein meal about an hour before his session with the therapist and still cannot remember the sounds, his auditory memory is poor and extra B_6 (100 to 200 mg) might be tried.

In Level V are found the severe hyperactive and genetically dyslectic children. These latter come from families in which most of the males have a lifelong problem of dyslexia, or else these children suffered some insult at birth that caused a defect in the integrative area of the cortex. We do what we can. Medication may help (Ritalin®, amphetamines, Cylert®). Some of these children manage by learning their lessons aurally from tapes and "writing" their papers into a recorder. The information goes from the ears to the brain to the tongue. Schools usually prefer the eyes-brain-hand method, but we must try everything that allows success and the development of that precious self-image.

Epilepsy is the term applied to lapses of consciousness with or without motor activity, usually associated with abnormalities of brain waves as shown in the electroencephalogram (EEG). It is a frightening condition to lay people, who associate it with brain damage and general intellectual deterioration. It can be the result of injuries to the brain, although the seizures themselves are not considered injurious. The cause of the seizure is considered the problem.

A child of eighteen months seen recently was noted to have eyelid twitching, left-arm flexion, and head tilting when but a few days old. Big doses of phenobarbital and Dilantin made the condition worse. The parents consulted another physician, who discovered low calcium in the blood and in a hair sample. Within two weeks of 500 mg of calcium twice a day orally, the child became calm, relaxed, and seizure-free. She is now talking and walks with help, but she has trouble using her left arm and tends to lean to one side.

The mother's history was revealing in that she had a milk allergy and had avoided milk for years. The extra stress of the pregnancy must have exhausted her calcium so the baby was not getting enough. Low calcium can cause tetany (twitching muscles) and lead to convulsions.

Babies born of diabetic mothers may overproduce insulin because of the extra glucose floating about in the blood stream. At birth the baby's pancreas does not shut off its insulin production, and the resulting hypoglycemia may cause seizures.

In the 1950s some milk came on the market that was low in B_6, and some babies who were fed this milk exclusively developed seizures.

In general, seizures that occur soon after birth are the result of brain injury from a difficult delivery, a metabolic problem of the mother, an infection in the mother transmitted to the baby, or to a lack of oxygen due to prematurity, lung immaturity, or partial strangulation by the umbilical cord.

Supportive measures for the at-risk baby include oxygen, blood, correction of acid-base imbalances and low blood sugar, antibiotics for infections, maintenance of correct body temperature, search for and removal of blood clots on the brain, and adequate feeding with breast milk if possible. These babies should have vitamin supplements under the assumption that the mother's diet was somehow inadequate or the baby would not be in this precarious condition.

The calcium, magnesium, and blood-sugar levels, at least, should be checked, since these, if low, will precipitate seizures in the compromised infant. If an infection is present, vitamin C should be administered (intravenously is preferable) in 50-to-100-mg doses several times a day along with whatever antibiotic is used.

Antiseizure medication would seem appropriate if all the metabolic, traumatic, anoxic, and infection problems have been attended to, remembering that anticonvulsants are only treating the symptoms. Extra B complex vitamins orally or by injection (up to 10 to 50 mg of each of the Bs, especially B_6, would be prudent since the baby has experienced stress from the delivery and the seizures and probably now has exhausted adrenal glands).

The older infant or young child who develops seizures with the onset of fever is not considered an epileptic. These are febrile seizures, believed to be caused by the stress of the sudden rise in temperature heralding a disease (usually viral in origin).

Most doctors put these children on a daily dose of phenobarbital to prevent a recurrence. This is standard treatment, but the fact of the infection suggests some lack of a nutrient or inadequate vitamin C in the tissues that allowed the invasion of the germ or virus. These febrile seizures are alarming, especially for the child's parents, and it is difficult to believe they do no harm, so the prophylactic phenobarbital seems wise.   (Giving it at the beginning of the sickness has been found to be ineffective.)

Some nocturnal seizures have been assumed to be due to a fall of blood sugar during sleep that sets off an "irritable focus" in the brain.   These may go unrecognized except by a suspicious family who notes a groggy child, a wet bed, a bitten tongue on a morning following some dietary excess or stress of some kind.

Some ecologically oriented doctors now feel that although hereditary factors and/or cerebral injuries can allow convulsions to appear, their severity and frequency may be assuaged by supernutrition. A neurologist would be the proper person to do the initial workup, with a physical exam, blood tests, and an electroencephalogram or brain scan.   A prescription for medication and arrangements for follow-up care are usually necessary.   A few additional things should be kept in mind.   Internal hormonal control keeps the concentrations of calcium and magnesium at fairly constant levels despite fluctuations in intake.   Hair analysis can reflect storage excesses or deficiencies.

Some growing children, especially meat-eaters, may be low in B_6, a deficiency of which may cause an irritable nervous system.

Low manganese levels often are seen in epileptics.

Low or rapidly falling blood sugar can trigger seizures in almost anyone.   The electroencephalogram taken before breakfast may give a different reading than one taken afterward.

Cerebral allergy always should be kept in mind when any odd behavior is noticed.   An allergy to corn, milk, wheat, potatoes, chocolate, eggs, drugs, additives, food colors, and the like should be suspected if a child (or adult) has seizures, sudden bouts of temper, extreme mood swings, fits of depression, or episodes of intense hyperactivity.   These unexpected outbursts may occur due to an overload of unfavorable factors (a stress occurs when the blood sugar is low, and the allergen has been consumed, and the victim didn't get his required sleep the night before). Some seizures are triggered by light hitting the eyes at a certain angle or by a certain kind of music.

The treatment of seizures is a complicated medical specialty and anyone so afflicted should be seeing a qualified practitioner, but a well-nourished brain is less likely to send out seizure-provoking electrical waves. The hopeful thought is that as the brain matures the child will be less prone to seizure.

Exhaustion (fatigue) for no good reason can be a nutritional problem, sometimes easily corrected. Before the child (or adult) is labeled lazy or suffering from mononucleosis, a check for anemia is standard. If the circulating iron or hemoglobin is lower than normal for the age, a trial of iron supplement usually corrects the blood picture and restores energy. Just about any iron salt (ferrous sulfate, gluconate, and the like) will work, although an iron chelate will be absorbed better with less chance of constipation or stomachache. Taking vitamin C (100 to 500 mg) with the iron enhances its absorption. The iron supplement should be continued for one to three months to assure adequate buildup of the iron storage in the body. Some attention should be paid to the reason for the anemia. In the one- to three-year age group it is usually the ingestion of too much cow's milk. Breast-fed babies rarely get iron-deficiency anemia.

Copper in small amounts is necessary for the proper formation of hemoglobin. A woman recently found that her body could not keep pace with her mind. After a reasonably normal day about the house, she would become exhausted at about 4:30 P.M. "I'll just take a short, refreshing nap before the family gets home." She would awaken at 7:00 A.M. She tried vitamins and the Prevention Diet and could keep going until 5:30 P.M. A psychiatrist felt she was retreating from reality because she was unable to emulate her mother. Someone checked her hair for minerals and found she was low in copper. A week after adding one mg of copper to the Prevention Diet and the vitamins, she was able to stay alert and comfortable until 9:30 P.M. She also discovered that her family wasn't all that exciting.

Exhaustion can be the result of an excess of some minerals, or an imbalance at least. In general, too much calcium and magnesium have a sedative effect. Low levels of chromium, selenium, and molybdenum can be associated with fatigue. Low thyroid function is usually associated with sluggishness; it is sometimes difficult to determine whether this is related to low blood sugar, insufficient stimulation from the pituitary, thyroiditis, or an iodine deficiency. A morning armpit temperature that consistently stays about 97° would warrant a trial of thyroid replacement hormone. Depression due to poor nutrition or psychological factors is usually accompanied by fatigue. Any drug can be a drag on the body. Carbon monoxide poisoning, fluoride in the water, food additives—the list of fatigue makers is endless.

A Level I child, if he gets his required amount of sleep and proper dream time, will awaken refreshed, alert, and cheerful. He will maintain this even level of responsiveness, being neither hyper- nor hypoactive unless bored or overstimulated. Usually after age five years he can abandon his nap without interfering with this evenness of energy. Under age five years, his naps would refresh him back to his presleep level.

In Level II, a child may have to take an extra ten minutes in the morning to get going. He may drop off to sleep if forced to sit still watching a boring movie. But he is generally responsive and can keep up with his peer group.

In Level III he is tired and grouchy. He may appear pale and sunken-eyed. He is reluctant to join friends in games. He is not refreshed in the morning after adequate sleep for his age. A minimum workup would include a test for anemia and infection (the sedimentation rate is standard). Swollen glands or a hidden urinary infection may be draining his energy. A diabetes test is usually thrown in. A review of his diet should be done to determine if he is ingesting refined carbohydrates or some food additives, colorings, or flavorings that might be related to his low energy levels. This would be especially helpful if he tends to be low in the morning after eating some sugary dessert before bedtime. Less than optimum growth from year to year, associated with fatigue, may suggest a thyroid evaluation or wrist x-ray for bone age. Heart defects that produce fatigue usually are associated with blue discoloration of nails and lips. If nothing causative is found and the doctor says he is all right, the Prevention Diet plus vitamins and a trial elimination of the child's favorite food should do something to elevate the energy level. A few weeks spent in another house or at a motel may be revealing, since allergens in the heating or cooking systems of the family house could be the problem. Do not overlook the depressing effects of psychological factors. Institutionalized children who are receiving little love and stimulation appear sluggish and withdrawn; children need positive strokes.

In Levels IV and V a child should get more extensive testing of brain and endocrine functions. A hair analysis of exhausted people frequently reveals low mineral levels and evidence of poor adrenal-gland function. Poisoning by lead and other heavy metals can cause fatigue. The five- or six-hour glucose tolerance test usually will be abnormal. Allergic testing may reveal an unsuspected pollen or food sensitivity. A controlled fast of three to four days might help.

Fatigue can follow from chronic stress and its accompanying low blood sugar. Chronic stress can lead to chronic disease, in large part explained by the exhausted adrenal glands continually having to get cortisone out into the blood stream. If the adrenals are not provided with the raw materials to continue to function, some disease process will take over. The patient and his doctor are so busy treating the symptoms and signs of this diagnosed condition that they forget to do anything about the pooped-out adrenals. The Stress Formula is the first step in the rehabilitation.

Fainting is supposed to happen mainly to women in distress. But anyone can keel over. If one feels faint, then faints and recovers promptly when horizontal, it tends to rule out epilepsy, since epileptics usually have no warning. Postural hypotension due to insufficient blood supply to the brain is the basic mechanism that causes the faint, but *that* could be due to emotional trauma, food allergies, low blood sugar, all of this aggravated by anemia, low thyroid function, or a stomachache that diverts the blood supply to the abdomen.

If one habitually drops to the floor on leaping out of bed in the morning, some attention must be paid to the bedtime snack. Obviously extra protein would be wise.

A pregnant woman who feels faint must change her diet, since the physiological anemia produced by the increase in blood volume will not oxygenate all her brain cells, and if she is not properly nourished a mild hypoglycemia will tip her over.

Some women faint from severe menstrual cramps that seem to send all the blood to the pelvis. Checking for anemia and taking extra calcium should stop this by the next period.

Some sensitive people faint with only minor injuries, which would suggest that they cannot screen out unimportant stimuli.

Fears in children seem completely irrational to the adults who observe a frightened child. We can explain, cajole, remonstrate, and be firmly supportive, but the child is rigidly locked into his belief: "There is an evil person in the dark there," "I will die if I ride in the car," "Something awful will happen if I go to school," "This food is poisoned." These fixed ideas usually crop up at age three to five years and may persist for years or even for a lifetime. The fear may have been triggered by a real event—a fire the child has witnessed, or a car accident, or some very traumatic, realistic television show or movie. It is logical to assume that something was perceived simultaneously with a heavy secretion of adrenalin; the adrenalin makes the perception scary, giving rise to that feeling of impending doom.

If your child says he is scared to go to bed, he may be telling you that he is secreting a lot of adrenalin. If he has never before felt frightened by something in his bedroom; if there is a nightlight on; if you have been loving, supportive parents; and if there is no good reason for his phobia, you can do two things. Check his pulse and see if it is unusually rapid (maybe twenty beats per minute over his usual rate), and write down what he had to eat in the previous few hours. Some sugary snack or a food to which he is sensitive may be the cause of the falling blood sugar that triggers the release of the adrenalin.

A Level I child has reasonable fears: busy streets, playing with matches, guns, knives. He can be easily reasoned with and reassured about new events. After age three he enjoys a visit to the doctor's office. He doesn't like the idea of the dentist, but of course he never has had any real tooth problems.

In Level II, a child could be reassured with explanations and charts and a "dry run" (seeing the school or hospital before beginning school or going in for an operation). He is occasionally frightened, but he also is thrilled by the excitement of scary stories or movies. He does not dwell on things. He could be frightened if left alone in a strange place (up to age seven). Simply being loving and sympathetic may be sufficient to allay his fears.

A Level III child has some new fear almost daily (*see* Anxiety, above). He is usually a child who needs (or needed as an infant) some rhythmical activity to become comfortable. His diet should be changed, and if that is not enough, he should receive the Stress Formula and probably extra calcium. If his fears are more acute at bedtime or through the night, his diet from lunch to bedtime should be changed. If his problem is facing the world in the daytime, his bedtime snack or breakfast may be triggering the adrenalin.

A Level IV child might have his fear of animals defused by showing him a picture of the animal at a safe distance while he is eating or being held comfortably in his parent's arms. The picture is moved closer each day for weeks until it is close to him but does not trigger his alarm button. Then daily exposure to the live animal is started, first at a distance and then gradually closer. It is immediately removed from view if anxiety appears.

Fear of the dark should be handled with lights and a flashlight for the child's own use. There is no way we can live in our child's body and experience the panic he is going through; we must assume it is very real. Parents should be sympathetic and supportive. Don't throw the child into his "fear" to show him it is groundless—he may never trust you again. Intellectually he may accept the fact that it is irrational, but the fear is nonetheless very real.

In Level V some tranquilizers may be necessary to calm the child so he can handle the dark, the water, the school, the trip, the crowd, and so on, until he can come to terms with it. Psychotherapy may be necessary to work out the details of the cause of the phobia. Hypnosis may be needed.

Habits of rhythmical rocking, sucking, tapping, banging, twisting, rubbing, shaking, chewing, and picking frequently drive even the calmest parents to lash out in anger and frustration. We have all heard it said, and grandparents sometimes reinforce the idea, that children who suck or rock are nervous and insecure and, of course, will grow up to be neurotics or alcoholics.

The monumental work of Lee Robins, *Deviant Children Grow Up*, has dispelled this idea with statistics showing that children who do these things grow up to be reasonably normal adults and that their children often have the same rhythmical habits. Perhaps that is why we may be unhappy to discover our own child doing something we did as children; it must revive an old memory of our parents' disgust with us for acting immaturely.

An insecure child may appear frightened and withdrawn and may need some rhythmical activity to calm his feelings. The child may indeed feel insecure because he perceives a scary world. It may be that his world is a threatening one and he has every reason to retreat or rock to block it out. But how do we explain this behavior when the home and the parents provide love, support, and security? It must be that the child is suffering from a stimulus overload. Because screening abilities are inadequate, he is unable to exclude extraneous sensory stimuli; his neocortex simply cannot handle all that arrives at that level. He tries to retreat or hide and cannot, so he "invents" a new stimulus that makes him feel comfortable; he is applying the principle of the gate theory to block out unwanted or noxious input. (If one nerve pathway is in use, another adjacent one will become blocked.)

All humans try for comfort. Experts in the electroencephalographic field report that we are the calmest when we are in alpha waves. These particular brain waves are present in the electroencephalogram when we are comfortable, secure, but still alert and aware. Beta waves are of a different length and are associated with irritability, touchiness, and vague feelings of discomfiture or danger. Infants find that the rhythmical motions they perform will send sensory messages to the cortex that are more comforting than those they are already receiving; hence they move themselves from beta waves to alpha waves. By rocking or sucking, they shut off or gate the undesirable stimuli.

Because these children need to do this, it accomplishes nothing to make a child stop one activity, since he will soon take up another. I have seen children who, on being forced to stop sucking their thumbs, merely picked up another habit like rocking or bottom-clutching.

We can let it go and assume the child will outgrow the habit, knowing these rhythmical activities have no predictive significance unless we label the child "bad" because of them. Most of them quit when their peer group calls them "Baby." We can be loving and supportive in the meantime and find alternatives (drums, toys, abacus, knitting, weaving, crayons, paint, mud, clay, sewing, basket-weaving—busy work). But if a parent says frequently enough "Only bad children suck their thumbs, and they grow up to be bums or alcoholics," the child will very possibly fulfill the prophecy.

A friendly dentist can sometimes motivate a child (usually after age six or seven) to discipline the sucking habit by giving him suitable reminders and rewards. It is amazing to most parents how some children will give up a cherished seven-year habit when an "authority" says it must be done. Hypnosis, too, may work.

A biochemical approach also can be effective before the habit becomes a way of life. Recently a feisty little five-year-old gave up her handshaking and waving habit after a few days of nutritious diet, including calcium and magnesium. She had been drinking plenty of milk but was either not absorbing it or had an allergy to it (or to something in it) that made her uncomfortable, so that the world seemed too close and threatening.

A Level I child might suck on thumb or fingers to keep hunger pains away. He might rock or twist because of a dirty diaper.

In Level II he would suck on a thumb and rock for five to fifteen minutes to get to sleep. He could easily be distracted from these rhythmical tension-relievers with calm speech, music, eating, games, or friends. New situations would remind him to revert to his old habits.

If he arrives at Level III, he will need to continue his efforts to keep the world at a safe distance for years—probably until age five to seven. He is more likely to be sensitive to noises, sights, and new situations. He clings alternately to reliable parents and to soft fuzzy toys. He drags bits of blanket or towels with him everywhere. He is more comfortable if his daily routine is not varied; he will have insomnia if the family moves. He is sensitive and ticklish and frequently has allergies; runny nose and bowels complicate his life. The B vitamins and calcium and magnesium would be in order. Comfort, love, and a quiet room in which to retreat are important supports.

A Level IV rocker, sucker, or twister needs help as soon as he is recognized. His life is miserable; he cannot relax because he is threatened on all sides by sights, sounds, smells, feelings. The possibility of autism may be considered, since eye contact makes him feel as if pins are being thrust into him. He may stiff-arm anyone who attempts to cuddle him. He is so busy sucking on his whole hand that it must be pulled away to get a nipple into his mouth. He sits on the edge of new and pleasant activities, sucking, rocking, twisting. Any pressure to participate is met with wild stiffening, flailing, fighting. Heavy doses of tranquilizers may not be enough to get him to relax and enjoy life. He is a prime candidate for school phobia.

Many children in this category seem bent on self-destruction. They bang their heads on the wall, bruising themselves and forming calcium deposits that make some foreheads pointed like a streamlined jet. Some will twist and pull out bunches of hair (trichotillomania), so that they appear to have ringworm of the scalp. A few strange children hit their faces with their fists or pinch off bits of skin. Some are considered autistic or retarded when they do this; it is difficult to believe this self-destructive action is psychogenic. Many are helped with cod-liver oil drops (500 to 1000 units vitamin D per day), which suggests a calcium deficiency.

In Level V, the child may need psychiatric care, foster-home placement, drugs, hair analysis, and a brain-wave test. Lead poisoning, high copper storage, and low zinc, calcium, or magnesium levels have been associated with these severe, unrelenting tension-relieving actions. One to two grams of niacinamide and 500 to 800 mg of pyridoxine are frequently helpful.

Headaches in children are usually the harbinger of "that virus that's going around." The virus in the brain cells causes a generalized swelling, and this stretching of the sensitive lining membranes causes the pain. The headache in this situation should be generalized. If the child is able to move about and if his neck and back are flexible (if he can "kiss his knees"), it would be permissible to load him up with vitamin C (maybe 500 to 1000 mg every hour or two), give him aspirin (1 grain per ten pounds of body weight every three to four hours), and a comfortable hot bath. If the temperature can be temporarily relieved, one might safely wait for developments.

Headache, fever, stiff neck, and convulsions are symptoms of a life-threatening meningitis or encephalitis. Do not fool around with the "too little and too late." Get the child to the hospital immediately.

Headaches located over cheeks, forehead, between the eyes, or at the very top of the head suggest sinus congestion, and when associated with a cold or green discharge from the nose, with or without fever, they may be worth treating with an antibiotic. Sinusitis is an infection, but an allergy allows the infection to become superimposed. Apparently the bacteria grow easily on the mucus produced by the allergy. Since the sinuses are not completely developed until after ages six to ten years, headaches due to sinus infection are rare in infancy and childhood, but the Stress Formula should be initiated. Milk allergy plays a significant role here; however, if all of the above are associated with sneezing and nose-rubbing, then an inhalation allergy would be more likely to set off the chain of events.

Stress can certainly cause a headache, but the frequency and location can be mimicked by food allergy or cerebral allergy or low blood sugar or migraine or a vascular headache. A nerve pinched by a spastic muscle in the back of the neck may cause a back-of-the-head headache, but falling blood sugar may cause the muscle to go into spasm to begin with. The idea is to keep the blood sugar so even and constant that the stresses of life will not depress this level to a point where the cerebral vessels dilate and cause the pounding.

A Level I child has never experienced a headache, except once when he walked into a door.

In Level II, the occasional headache (two or three a year) is associated with some disease or hangover (the day after Easter chocolate).

Most of us are in Level III for headaches, where infections, allergies, stress, pollution, food additives, fluorescent light may all combine with falling blood sugar to make the brain or cerebral blood vessels dilate. Each time there is a headache, someone should write down the foods, additives, and flavors that have been consumed in the preceding six to twelve hours. A morning headache might be due to the dish of chocolate ice cream consumed at bedtime, although the anticipation of a stressful test might make it worse. (I thought my Thursday-evening headaches were the result of the stress of my partner's afternoon off, but when I took the time to eat a better lunch, no headache appeared. If I eat white cheese and old-fashioned peanut butter on whole wheat bread I'm all right until 7:00 P.M., but processed luncheon meat on white bread for lunch will give me a nagging headache by 4:00 P.M. The point is, one can handle stress if the brain is properly nourished.) The nibbling diet, no sugar, and the Stress Formula would be appropriate for those in Level III.

In Level IV, the victim is usually in the migraine category, had cyclic vomiting as a child, can't stand fluorescent light or bright sunlight, takes aspirin almost daily, and runs the risk of moving up to aspirin with codeine or something stronger. If the antistress program has been tried for at least a month with no success, a review of the diet would be wise, with the idea in mind that the culprit is an allergy to some food that is frequently eaten and enjoyed. Usually it is found to be a favorite: milk, coffee, chocolate, corn, nuts, beef, potatoes, wheat, eggs and the like. A three-day fast might give some insights; if one feels terrific on the third or fourth day, foods are reintroduced every few days until the headache returns. I recall a ten-year-old boy, the son of a dairy farmer, who had incapacitating headaches due to you-know-what. An ounce of beer or a swallow of red wine can put some people on the floor with a screamer in just two hours. In general, if caffeine (as in coffee), tea, No-doz, Empirin, or Anacin makes the aspirin work better, it suggests a vascular headache, a low-blood-sugar headache, or a migraine—but all these could be related to allergies. Much nausea and vomiting associated with the headache suggests it is migraine, possibly related to low blood sugar. The victims are people who cannot get the sugar out of storage in the liver; the resulting acidosis from fat mobilization and the dilation of the cerebral blood vessels in trying to increase the nutrients to the brain put them in bed in a dark room for a day. Children with stomachaches frequently have headaches as adults. Some families don't know what a headache is. In general, sugar causes thin, hyperactive people to have headaches and fat, quiet people to feel tired, heavy, and hungry. Low thyroid might allow a mild fullness to become a headache.

Level V headache victims are very sick with headaches and need a neurological workup to rule out space-occupying lesions (blood clots, tumors, cysts, infections). An EEG and brain scan might be included. If "organic" lesions can be ruled out, we are back to stress, psychic causes, allergies, migraine, hypoglycemia. A headache is Mother Nature's way to tell you that something is wrong with your head, your food, your life.

Hyperactivity is activity increased to a degree noticeable by an observer. It is only a problem if the active person is put down because of it. If the parents, teachers, and peer group have to say to the active one "Sit down," "Get out of there," "Stop doing that," and these are the only things the child hears from his environment, he may then develop a bad self-image. About 20 to 30 percent of the population seems to be susceptible to increased activity when under stress from increased sensory stimuli (large classroom, some fluorescent light, nonionizing radiation), falling blood sugar (from ingestion of sugar or allergenic foods), psychogenic causes (unaccepting environment or poor support systems), and metabolic problems (lead poisoning, inadequate B complex vitamins, low calcium, low magnesium, low thyroid).

Genetic factors are important; whole families may be leaping about, staying up late, all talking and jiggling at once. They may think that a relatively calm child is sick.

The Level I child is calm despite noise and excitement, can fall asleep almost everywhere, and can even eat some junk food without getting excited. He rarely sucks his thumb or bounces his leg up and down.

A Level II hyperactive child seems to be able to turn activity on and off as needed; he has self-control. In a noisy, distracting classroom he might be the last one to begin spinning around, and he only does this because he wants peer-group acceptance.

In Level III he is noticeably restless only in the supermarket, the classroom, the circus, or at noisy parties. He is cheerful enough to smile his way out of these situations when someone calls his attention to his movements. He is clever enough to get his work done. The teacher says about this child "He could do better" or "I know he knows it, but he won't put it down on paper." He could be diagnosed as having "situational hyperactivity"; the problem is not present when he is at home with a single parent or at school alone with the teacher after classes. It appears with stress, a big classroom, or a tough teacher. He is hyper with one teacher but not another. He is worse in the open classroom and does better in a smaller, structured classroom with a teacher who is neither a martinet nor a do-whatever-you-want type. This Level III child may need medicine only on bad days or occasionally for only one teacher. He is a borderline case. The nutritional Stress Formula should allow him to function up to his potential—liking school, keeping up with his peers, and—of course—developing a good self-image.

If he slips into Level IV he may be developing a bad self-image and may be hating school, home, and people because his hyperactivity seems unrelated and inappropriate and he usually gets the bad strokes—the questions and commands. Life is a gyp; he feels cheated out of his birthright, a happy childhood. He is getting depressed and sulky because everything he does at home, on the playground, or in school is met negatively. School will make this child worse, but the early warning signs of insomnia, rhythmical habits, much sickness and many allergies, Jekyll-and-Hyde behavior should have alerted his parents to the need to remedy his disruptive behavior years earlier. Love is not enough; a little chemistry is needed. Before the child slips into Level V he should get extra calcium and magnesium as well as the Stress Formula; a search should be made for hidden sugar and chemicals (salicylates in foods) and for allergens in food, air, and water. An evaluation of the thyroid function and a hair analysis for the levels of stored minerals also might be needed.

It is difficult for me to accept the surprise of parents on learning of their child's hyperactivity in the stressful (to him) and distracting classroom. Certainly parents should be able to perceive the antecedents by age two or three. A two-year-old should be able to listen to a ten-minute story read by a loving parent without tearing about the room. A three-year-old should be able to sit and watch a fifteen-minute age-appropriate television program without having to stand on his head. You should be able to take a four-year-old grocery shopping with only five interruptions. A five-year-old should be able to attend kindergarten with his name, age, and address clearly in memory, and be able to sit still and attend to schoolwork for at least ten or fifteen minutes. At all these ages children should be able to laugh more than cry and be able to follow a few commands to completion. They should hear more compliments about their behavior than criticism.

If discovered in Level V, a hyperactive child usually needs remediation with stimulant drugs to slow him down. This motor-driven child is "off the wall" despite a calm, firm, loving environment; he needs no external stimuli to rev him up. He acts as if he has a hot cattle-prod in his rectum. A trial of Ritalin®, Dexedrine®, or Cylert® would be approprite to see if some calmness could be attained. His response would suggest the next reliable step. If a stimulant does quiet him, we know he has a fault in his neurobiochemical pathways and the suggested approaches for Level IV have not been pursued sufficiently. It also suggests that he is in a stressful situation that no nutritional formula will control (home breaking up; evil, frightening, punitive parents; overgraded in school; reading disability; sleeping in a small bed with two brothers who wet the bed; or something of the sort).

School counselors, psychologists, psychiatrists, social workers all may have to take a crack at this problem before the child is thrown out of school. Mellaril®, or Valium® may have to be tried. An EEG might reveal something treatable. The prenatal history might be helpful. These children usually were impoverished nutritionally long before birth and then experienced a traumatic or early birth, so that some sign of brain damage is associated with the hyperactivity.

Many of us who deal with these children find that B complex vitamin injections are helpful. B_6 in 200-to-500-mg doses may turn the trick. Often, big doses of calcium (1000 to 2000 mg per day) plus vitamin D (500 to 1000 units per day) will calm them. Extra zinc (50 to 90 mg per day) may be a partial answer. Foster care in a farm setting may break the vicious cycle.

Hyperventilation is rapid, deep respiration beyond that required for the oxygen needs of the body. It is considered a sign of anxiety and is usually associated with excess secretion of adrenalin and rapid pulse. A frightening thought might trigger an attack, but if it occurs without apparent warning, it may be caused by nutritional factors or stress. The triggering chemical event seems to be the fall in blood sugar caused by the excess insulin that results from the ingestion of sugar or an allergen. The adrenalin produced by falling blood sugar tells the body that something awful is happening. The body breathes deeply, the heart races, the pupils dilate (the fight-or-flight mechanism).

The excessive breathing without simultaneous muscle use reduces the carbon dioxide level in the blood, the blood shifts slightly to the alkaline side, the calcium ions are less soluble, and muscle-twitching and even fainting and convulsions follow. Here is another example of a chemical event appearing to be a psychiatric one.

A diet change seems appropriate, including an increase in calcium ingestion (see Chapter 2). This explanation does not rule out psychogenic causes, since people who are susceptible to hyperventilation usually are in need of psychiatric support. It simply indicates that if touchy people are well nourished, they may need fewer supportive measures.

Hypoglycemia is low blood sugar; it implies that the pancreas has overreacted to the glucose floating about in the blood stream by excreting more than enough insulin to get the blood sugar back to a normal level. Some sensitive people react to slight changes in their glucose level by secreting adrenalin; this makes their heart beat faster and makes them feel fearful or anxious that something terrible is about to happen. Others respond with antisocial, animalistic behavior. Apparently, the conscience in the higher reaches of the brain flicks out if the brain is not adequately and consistently nourished. If the conscience or super-ego area of the cortex is not nourished properly, it cannot monitor or control the animal or selfish lower centers. Some people develop headaches, asthma, hay fever, arthritis, stomachache—the so-called psychosomatic illnesses. The low blood sugar allows that person's genetic weakness to surface.

Insomnia manifests itself in two ways: in one, the child (or adult) cannot fall asleep; in the other, the victim awakens after one to five hours of sleep and can't get back to sleep. Although psychogenic factors are frequently given as the basis of insomnia, attention given to the neurochemical factors involved in sleep frequently solves the problem. It is important to control insomnia because the child who is up at night and wandering about looking for food or wanting to crawl into his parents' bed is more likely to become battered. The feisty, sensitive, touchy, goosey, talkative, ticklish, easily spooked child has trouble relaxing and falling asleep. Many have a ritual at bedtime, and if one step of the ritual is left out, the whole procedure must be repeated until it is just right: Brush teeth, say prayers, place toys and dolls in exactly the right place, have a story read, kiss both cheeks, say "nightie-night" three times—this may be just the minimum. Don't let the child feel it is silly; we all need these reassurances that we are cared for and that life will go on.

But where do we draw the line? Children all have different needs, but if the ritual gets longer, more complicated, and repetitious, maybe the child is pulling a deal, or maybe he perceives that his world is slipping—and maybe it is. If after much soul-searching you conclude that the environment you are providing is secure and supportive, then the child's rituals may mean that he is asking for limits or that his perceptions are askew. In either case, the Stress Formula and extra calcium might allow the nights to be easier. It might be worthwhile to compare the evening pulse with the afternoon pulse; an evening rate of 10 to 20 beats per minute higher *might* suggest a food allergy or a sugary food for supper that is stimulating the child and making it impossible for him to relax at bedtime. It is amazing how a piece of protein (meat, cheese, fish, egg, nuts) instead of a dish of ice cream about a half hour before bedtime allows the child to relax, say "nightie-night," and pop off to sleep. It also might make it easier if you call the child's bluff and, after ten minutes of fooling around at bedtime, say, "Okay! That's enough. Get into bed and go to sleep!" The child's new perception is "I feel more secure when I have rules to follow." A well-nourished brain allows for more accurate perceptions of the environment.

One of the most common calls pediatricians get concerns night wakefulness. The child seems to settle down easily and cheerfully at a reasonable time in the evening; he sleeps one to five hours and then is up and screaming, wandering, crying, moving from bed to bed, having a night terror, falling out of bed, urinating in the wastebasket—obviously not having a peaceful night's sleep. He will snuggle between the parents because of the monsters in his bed. This nocturnal restlessness is often called a habit, but we are now convinced that the awakening is due to a biochemical problem and the habit is what the child does once up and out of bed. (*See* Night terrors, below.)

A Level I child will go to bed willingly (although not always cheerfully) when asked. When he awakens, which is rare and usually due to gas or a full bladder, he settles right down again with a "Sorry I had to bother you." He rouses easily and cheerfully in the morning.

In Level II, he did not sleep through as an infant until he was two months old, probably because he was growing so fast he could not eat enough to carry him from 7:00 P.M. to 7:00 A.M. He would cry out occasionally at night between ages one and three years, but by the time the parents had reached the bedside, he was sound asleep. It was probably gas going around an intestinal corner or the passage of salty urine over a tender diaper rash.

The Level III child has to rock the bed or suck his thumb as part of the going-to-sleep routine. Putting the mattress on the floor spares everyone the noise of the crib ricocheting from wall to wall. This child needs to nurse or have a bottle at bedtime; he will awaken between midnight and 3:00 A.M. for months (and years), have about ten sucks and then return to a deep sleep. Is this habit? It would depend on the definition. Some doubt would be cast on the habit theory if the child sleeps through when one or more of the following measures are tried: (1) If he is on the bottle, making the bedtime bottle undiluted (dangerous to do all the time because of the heavy mineral load presented to the kidneys); (2) giving a protein feeding at bedtime, in case the wakefulness is due to falling blood sugar (a half to a whole jar of strained veal or lamb); (3) giving 500 to 1000 mg of calcium (dolomite, bone meal, or calcium gluconate) at bedtime with or without vitamin D (500 to 1000 units as cod-liver oil)—especially good for the child who needs to suck or rock to get to sleep or the older child who has muscle cramps, shin splints, or growing pains in the middle of the night; (4) changing the milk from cow's to goat's or soybean if on the bottle, and having the mother stop cow's milk if she is breast-feeding; (5) eliminating prescription vitamins that have additives, sugar, color, and fluoride; (6) and, of course, treating the child for the ubiquitous pinworms.

In spite of all of above, if he slips into Level IV, his whole life pattern must be reevaluated. Stress and allergies are the most difficult to trace, since we all react differently to them. Mold in the wall, some stuffing in a toy animal, or some foods previously thought to be safe could be stimulants (such as corn, potatoes, beef, wheat, eggs, chocolate). A few vitamin B complex shots (painful) might be revealing. If he is calmer, he needed them; if he is more hyperactive and restless, then the B vitamins released histamine, a stimulant to the brain, and he almost surely needs calcium and magnesium. A hair analysis would be appropriate at this time. Usually it reveals low levels of those two minerals. Lead levels may be up; zinc and copper and chromium may be up. A brain-wave test (sleeping) may show some odd paroxysms. Taking the temperature in the first waking minutes might tell something about the thyroid. We assume that your doctor has searched for urinary infections, low-grade throat and gland infections, and intestinal disorders; a complete blood count and sedimentation rate should have revealed something treatable before the parents hear the verdict "It must be psychogenic."

Twenty-five to 50 mg of zinc and 1 to 5 mg of manganese daily can be dramatic to induce calmness and natural sleep. Tryptophan, an amino acid, 500 mg, can produce drowsiness.

Irritability is an early warning sign of impending surliness, unruliness, and perhaps aggressive behavior. If the onset is abrupt, the safest thing to do would be to assume that the child is coming down with that virus that is going around. Do not wait; quadruple the vitamin C intake. An adult might take 1000 mg of C every hour if he has that all-over creepy feeling and a scratchy throat. A child may not be able to communicate that he feels this way, and by the time the flu symptoms are obvious the next day, the vitamin therapy is less reliable.

If a child displays the kicking-in-the-front-door syndrome after school, assume there was a birthday party or he traded his nutritious lunch for a bag of marshmallows. Before you even talk to him, get some protein down his throat plus a couple of big B complex vitamins and wait twenty to thirty minutes. *Then* ask him what happened at school. Do not talk to his animal brain. If he suddenly reverts to his infantile tension-relieving sucking or rocking, get some calcium (dolomite, bone meal) into him. Try a hot bath with the water running (this produces soothing negative ions).

If you haven't headed it off, the problem should show itself the next day: a cold, earache, vomiting, diarrhea, cutting a tooth, hives, hay fever, an asthma attack, gas, and so on. Call a doctor for some specific therapy but continue the vitamin program suited for the condition.

Jekyll-Hyde behavior displayed by sensitive children (or adults) is usually a diagnostic clue that a nutritional fault or some stress has interfered with the proper functioning of the neocortex and its contained conscience. If the humane parts of the brain are not constantly supplied with oxygen, amino acids, glucose, and the like, the subhuman areas will take over, and (depending upon genetic factors) aggressiveness, depression, paranoia, selfishness, impulsiveness, or some antisocial behavior will be manifest. This animal response cannot be dealt with, controlled, or treated. Attempts at behavior modification are close to pointless when there is no humane and logical communication possible with the subject. When the Dr. Jekyll part of the brain is functioning again it may be able to have insight into the previous disturbing behavior, but insights are impossible when the animal brain is in control (*see* Aggression, above, and Mood swings, below).

   Lying is so typical of the four- to five-year-old that we usually just call it "story-telling." The child is testing out the magic of words and experiments with statements like "There is a lion in the front yard." (Better check; he may be telling the truth.) However, if lying becomes a way of life and the child needs to do this to cover up his shortcomings, it suggests either that he has developed a bad concept of himself or that he really perceives this distortion as the explanation of his action.

   "How did the candy wrapper get under the bed?" you ask. "The dog put it there." The child probably put it there, but he cannot quite remember because his blood sugar was so low when he did it that the whole episode is as vague as the dream he had three nights ago. It is impossible to punish the animal brain that was responsible, and it seems to do no good to get mad at the neocortex since it was not "present" when the event took place. Even a lie detector won't get a reading on this one.

   This kind of lying is hard to treat, because the child feels no guilt or remorse or insight when confronted with witnesses

and overwhelming evidence that he was culpable. It is anal-
ogous to the chronic alcoholic's confabulation. Planning the
diet to prevent blood sugar dips should prevent recurrences.
The child also needs some strengthening of and rewards for
the good parts of his personality. He needs to win in some
socially acceptable area.

Memory is required by all us living things so we won't
make the same stupid, painful mistakes over and over again.
We know from memory that two and two equal four, that fire
is hot, that knives are sharp.

Researchers and philosophers are trying to differentiate
between phylogenetic instincts (so-called race memory) and
learned responses. Learning waits on maturation, and maturation is partly an inborn timing mechanism and partly a nutri-
tion-based phenomenon.

Most of our built-in emotional responses reside in the
animal brain. Memory resides in the cortex and subcortex.
These areas file away memories from life (perhaps also from
the lives of our ancestors). Each stimulus that comes into our
cortex from the body and the environment sets up a "reverbera-
tive circuit" that stores that memory forever.

It is believed that imprints received during the day are
retained in short-term memory circuits in or near the cortex
and are moved during sleep to long-term memory storage
banks. Thus, sleep time clears the cortex for the next day's
events.

It has been found that B_6 is necessary to activate the enzyme that is responsible for this memory transfer. Try 50 to
100 mg of pyridoxine (B_6) at bedtime along with some protein
to test this out; you should notice that you can remember your
dreams better. If your dreams are exciting, funny, or sexy, it
may be worthwhile. If they are stupid, forget it. (Some wag
once suggested that dreaming is our natural state and we
awaken only to eat and go to the bathroom.)

Teachers tell us that some pupils act as if they were retaining much information for a period of time and then, as if a trap door opened, it all falls out of their brains and the data are simply lost forever. These nonretainers can profit by 50 to 100 mg of B_6 daily. Remedial reading teachers frequently see improvement in pupils' skills when nutritional snacks and B_6 are given an hour or so before a lesson. Retention of the memory of the sounds of the letters is essential to reading. The cortex must be lit for this high human function to be possible.

Mood swings are a variant of Jekyll-Hyde behavior (*see* above). If a person is depressed and noncommunicative upon arising in the morning and seems alert and responsive and cheerful two hours after breakfast, the previous evening's meal may have been at fault. Usually it turns out that a sugary dessert or a bowl of ice cream at bedtime has excited the body to over-produce insulin, thus forcing the blood sugar down. Daily or hourly fluctuations are almost always due to food, while monthly or yearly variations suggest the manic-depressive type of personality. In the latter situation, the patient becomes manic, restless, has trouble sleeping, takes on too many tasks for three to six months and then is normal or becomes the opposite: he sleeps a lot, gets nothing done, is quiet, depressed, and pessimistic. Psychiatrists are clever at diagnosing and treating this condition. Lithium almost always controls the symptoms.

If a child seems surly, negative, touchy, grouchy all the time, some screening for anemia, worms, lead poisoning, milk or other allergy must be done. Humans are basically cheerful and gracious. When they are not, usually it is because something is preventing this attitude from surfacing.

Multiple sclerosis is a chronic, slowly progressive neurological disease that causes weakness of various muscles scattered about the body. Double vision, a leaky bladder, difficulty in raising a foot, an area of the skin that feels numb, a lack of feeling for temperature in another area are the protean manifestations of this disease of unknown etiology. Some now feel that the disease is due to a chronic virus that slowly destroys nerve tissue. Dr. Frederick Klenner has been using mega doses of vitamin C and the B complex to halt the spread of the virus with some success.

The disease is rare in children, but the implications for treatment of infectious diseases with supernutrition is exciting. Perhaps fewer of us would develop multiple sclerosis in adulthood if childhood diseases were considered a stress and supernourishment with C and B vitamins was followed routinely.

Neuritis is an inflammation of a nerve. If a doctor makes a diagnosis of this or polyneuritis, usually rest and aspirin are recommended. Because nerve function is intimately involved with the B vitamins, it would be logical to provide them in large doses.

Night terrors are frightening episodes that awaken the whole household at about one in the morning. The victim, usually a child, awakens screaming, pupils large, heart rapid and pounding, hot sweat all over. There is no reasoning with the child, who seems to be in a daze. In about twenty minutes the episode is over and he is back to sleep. Most do not remember the episode in the morning.

Apparently the falling blood sugar triggered the release of adrenalin, and the adrenalin made a normal dream into a nightmare. Stress, excitement, or frightening television can do this, but the usual story is that the child does not go to bed unless he has a bowl of cereal or ice cream as a bribe. The sudden sharp rise in blood sugar stimulates the pancreas to squirt out rapidly a good supply of insulin to help get the glucose into storage.

The cure would be a snack of some protein at bedtime and the elimination of all sugar and non-nourishing foods. Calcium (1000 mg), magnesium (500 mg), and stress amounts of the B complex should help. (B vitamins *can* stimulate some people, however; *see* Insomnia, above, and Pinworms, p. 153).

Restless legs in children are related to such rhythmical habits as thumb-sucking and rocking. A proper amount of calcium and magnesium along with the Prevention Diet and B complex should slow down legs that keep bouncing up and down. (*See* Habits, p. 201.)

Legs that need to be constantly twisted and stretched may respond to vitamin E (400 to 1200 units per day). Vitamin E seems to be helpful when circulation is impaired, so E might be more useful for the elderly, and calcium for the young.

Running away is more frequent in girls than boys. Usually they are eleven to sixteen years old and feel depressed, alone, unloved, gypped, and restless. They usually are not running *to* something, only *away* from something, but they seldom know why they are running.

Almost all these young people are on a high-carbohydrate diet—at a time when they are growing rapidly. They are hungry all the time, and if not provided with proper nutrition, they soon get habituated to sugary junk food. When the blood sugar starts to bounce around, they become weak, sick, tired, confused, surly—like a disturbed hibernating animal.

They get the perception that they are being picked upon; they are paranoid at times. They run because their space bubble is collapsing.

When they are gone, they are gone, but we must play their game their way. We worry. We are scared. We feel guilty. We get mad. We pray. We call the police. The children usually show up, none the worst for wear. But we can never, never, make fun of this (until twenty years later), because it is a very important and serious part of growing up.

I am impressed by how many of these young people show an abnormal glucose tolerance. Because they are eating so poorly, they don't know what they are doing.

I wonder if a lawsuit filed by the parents of a runaway against candy machine companies or junk-food manufacturers might get people to take notice. This is serious business. These sugar purveyors are toying with *lives*—our children's lives.

School failure is common because of our system of education. In our fang-and-claw philosophy, there are winners and losers, and if the losers having nothing else going for them to make them feel good about themselves, they become the failures. These are the ones the teacher can identify as having educational dysfunction and who are brought to our office for treatment. Of course, when we move a loser up a couple of places in the pecking order of the class, there is another one to take his place. (At least, the child may be comforted by seeing that he is not the only loser.)

During the school conference, the parents must listen for key phrases: "I know he knows the work, but he won't put it on paper"; "He won't work up to his ability"; "Some days he has it; the next day it's gone." These would suggest that nutritional factors are a part of the explanation. The off-and-on phenomenon is the clue to fluctuating blood sugar; if ticklishness, carbohydrate craving, and sleep difficulties also are present, nutrition is the key factor in helping this particular child. If a doctor prescribed Ritalin®, Cylert®, or dextroamphetamine to control the hyperactive behavior, and the child is calmer, it suggests that the child is not producing enough of his own norepinephrine. This further indicates that the enzyme producing the norepinephrine is defective and a nutritional approach should be helpful. (*See* Attention Span, Dyslexia, Hyperactivity, Ticklishness, elsewhere in this chapter.)

Separation fear or anxiety is common and is to be expected at about eight to twelve months of age. Usually there is screaming and panic when the child sees the mother leave the room, even for a second. The assumption is that the child finally realizes he is not attached to the mother; he is really alone and vulnerable. Our usual reassurances to parents is that this is normal.

But this, like so many other traits, is on a continuum—some is normal, but a lot is too much. How does one decide? The rule might be: If it bothers the parents or interferes with the *fun* of child rearing, do something.

Because it is a mild and short-lived problem in breast-fed babies, it seems wise to nurse a baby well into and after the months when the condition is at its peak. Try to nurse beyond one year of age. Some doctors used to feel that the bonding of mother and child produced by the immediate close liaison after birth would make later separation more difficult. Just the opposite is true, however. Early bonding and breast-feeding apparently make the baby so secure and calm that he can relax and look on growing up and moving away from mother as a happy part of life. It suggests that the superior intake of calcium in the breast-fed baby may contribute to his calmness.

The separation cry is hard to ignore—especially if you are the parent of the panicky baby and have been told by the doctor to let the child scream it out. In general, consoling the child every time he cries tends to perpetuate the problem. Instead, try giving him extra protein and calcium about an hour prior to the walking-out-of-the-room time. It may help him to stay calm.

Shingles is an inflammation involving a nerve distribution. It is caused by a virus related to chicken pox. The B complex taken orally (or, better, by injection) will speed up the recovery. B_{12} injections are traditional, but all the Bs are important.

Shyness is a normal response for most of us in new situations. We expect shyness in our children in the first few days of nursery school. They may hold back and watch the other children, then when curiosity gets them going or because it looks like more fun than sitting on the sidelines, they move out and participate, but always keeping an escape in view.

A little shyness, though, may be life-saving. We know how accident-prone the hyperactive approacher can be. Above all, don't try to cure it by direct countermoves, like throwing a water-shy child into the lake for his first swimming lesson. We cannot live inside the child's body and experience the scary perceptions or feel the surging adrenalin. We have to assume he is shy because of overwhelming dysperception and an adrenalin-related feeling of impending doom. Attempts to explain away the phobia will only fall on a deaf dinosaur brain.

Time is on your side. Let the child slowly digest the world, his world, as he sees it. Assume his supersensitivity and inappropriate shyness are due to falling blood sugar, extra adrenalin, and a poorly operating filtering system for sensory stimuli. Assume he "sees" an elephant when you and I might only see an aardvark.

You can help him handle new situations by showing equanimity yourself, but also by serving him the Prevention Diet and the Stress Formula. A big piece of protein (nuts, fowl, egg, fish, meat, cheese) just prior to the new situation is appropriate for everyone. (Feed the soldiers just before the battle.)

Stealing is an antisocial activity related to lying, arson, and cheating and is considered something that a delinquent

might do. Hypoglycemia has been found in adults who shop-
lift. When the energy flowing through the blood vessels to
the brain of an individual falls to a level that prevents the conscience (superego) from functioning, the lower, animal centers assume control. In that area are "Gimme," "I'm better
than you," "Too bad; you lose." No sense of right and wrong
is down there; the devil takes over.

I asked a twelve-year-old-boy picked up for stealing a
television set from a home what he had eaten on the day he
did the theft. The only thing he had eaten was a bowl of
processed cereal with sugar at eight-thirty in the morning.
The crime occurred at 4:30 P.M. The circuits in his conscience
that store the message "Do not steal" were out, and his internal
social controls were nonoperative.

Every person picked up for inappropriate behavior
should have a diet review or a five-hour glucose tolerance
test. I have patients who light fires only when they miss breakfast. Protein snacks will keep their consciences alert enough
to oversee social behavior. Barbara Reed, probation officer in
Cuyahoga Falls, Ohio, says about 80% of her clients are nutritionally ill.

Temper is no doubt affected by genetic factors, insults
before and during birth, supportiveness of the environment,
and nutrition. (*See also* Aggression, Biting, Delinquency,
Mood swings, and Running away, above.)

If a child has an explosive temper, it may mean that he
is sick and cannot cope. If his temper outbursts are intermittent and his basic personality is cheerful and compliant, then
diet, additives, stress, or allergies might explain the attacks.

Ticklishness is a sign that a child (or adult) is stress-
prone. It correlates with the individual's conception of his
personal space. If one is very ticklish, his space bubble is con-
stricted and the world seems close, either in a threatening or

an overstimulating way. There are many ticklish people in the world and apparently many of them do very well. But a child who is hyperactive or a troublemaker or wakeful or allergic is more likely to come from the ranks of the very ticklish. Of the last thousand educational dysfunction cases I have seen, only two were not rated 3 or 4 on a ticklishness scale of 1 to 4.

It is suggested, as a test of ticklishness, that on the first day of school the teacher have all the children lie down supine on the floor and remain motionless as long as possible. She then slowly lowers a "tickle machine" on them (twenty or thirty feathers tied at intervals along a long rod). The child who breaks first with giggles, snorts, rolling, twisting is the one to watch or separate or tone down the environment for.

The condition is almost quantifiable and represents a defect in the structure or function of the limbic filtering system. The chemical responsible for this filtering appears to be norepinephrine, a stimulant; hence stimulant medications (Ritalin®, Cylert®, dextroamphetamine) all have a calming effect on the person so put together. They serve to enlarge his space bubble thus making him more comfortable and able to cope with stress.

But we also know what will help enzyme functions—protein snacks, B vitamins, calcium—and what has a calming effect on the nerve tissue.

Tics or twitches are muscle spasms; some people are prone to them, especially when under stress. Small groups of muscles around the eye or mouth will jerk spasmodically and often at the most embarrassing times. If they become more frequent during stress, the treatment is clear; remove the stress or take the Stress Formula.

Muscles depend on calcium to function properly; indeed, the condition of tetany is due to low calcium. Are tics the harbinger of tetany? Extra calcium stops these twitches in just a few hours.

Stress depletes calcium from the system. If people with tics cannot get out from under a stress, they should at least follow the whole program and the Stress Formula plus one gram of calcium per day.

Vandalism is an aspect of delinquent behavior. If a school has been pillaged for no good reason, the principal pulls a list of suspects out of his file. It is the ten to twenty pupils who are the school failures in the various classes. He knows who did it, and the vandals know why they did, but they usually have verbal expression problems so they won't communicate. If someone is made fun of and called stupid long enough, he will finally become depressed, run away, or fight back.

After all this seething hostility builds up in the adolescent, it requires only a slight trigger to set the charge off: a "lecture" from a hated teacher, a friend who didn't say hello, being dropped from the team for bad grades, then (you guessed it) a bottle of wine, a bag of candy, a load of ice cream, and the blood sugar falls and the little bit of remaining conscience in the neocortex is lost. The school, church, house, whatever, is gutted, kicked, burned, and often urinated upon.

We know what is behind this senseless property waste. The schools are trying, at least, to make the schools better. What is needed is for somebody to do something about the avalanche of junk food, which increasingly displaces nutritious food in the diets of these kids and disposes them to rampage.

□

No teacher should be required to teach a child who did not bring his brain to school; she cannot teach the animal limbic system. Every morning each pupil should report what his breakfast contained. If he had no protein and ate mainly carbohydrates, he should be sent home.

Afterword: How to Begin

I believe that the most important pathway to mental and physical health is the *conviction* that improvement is possible, no matter what the condition or the age of the person may be. Motivation must be present. In order to bring about change you must *believe* that you will feel better, or that you will look better, or that you will save money, or that anxiety will be reduced, or that the quality of life will be improved.

The parent who sets out to change his or her family's eating habits overnight is likely to meet loud and vigorous opposition. No one likes having favorite foods snatched away. These parents should not become discouraged. Instead, they should proceed gradually and play on the motivational theme. If you tell an adolescent to quit eating junk food so his school-work will improve, he is not likely to change. If you guarantee more stamina for sports and fewer pimples, you will probably get results.

What you are aiming for in your house is simplicity and effectiveness; if it is too complicated, it won't be done. Some

228

well-motivated adults can change habits overnight, but children may need a few months of subtle changes in diet to effect changes in body chemistry and sweet cravings. It might be wise to provide a junk-food night once a week or two so the child will not have withdrawal anger and depression. Shoring up the enzymes with extra B-complex vitamins at those times may prevent the symptoms from surfacing. If you know that you or your child is going to be tempted at a party, throw down two capsules before and after. (B complex can shorten or eliminate the hangover, as the Bs allow the liver enzymes to metabolize alcohol more efficiently.)

If you have never allowed your baby to experience the addictive taste of sugar in food, you will never have to experience with him the pain of withdrawal. We assume in the following example that you have been giving only breast (or bottle) milk for the first six to eight months of life. Now, boredom, teeth, and in-law pressure have pushed you to try some solids.

At age six to ten months, increasing gradually, give one to ten teaspoons of oatmeal one or two times a day. Sprinkle wheat germ on this, and ever so slowly over the weeks stir in brewer's yeast powder. It may be cut with your own home-made apple sauce. After eight to ten months give this solid first and let the baby decide how much milk he wants afterward. If you are not sure that he is getting at least 500 to 800 mg of calcium, add enough bone meal or dolomite powder to the basic cereal to correct this possible deficiency (especially if he is a rocker, a thumb sucker, or is wakeful).

Cottage cheese pureed with fruit could be added at about ten to eleven months. Carrot, celery, and beet juice could be the next addition or use these vegetables steamed and mashed. Three to six meals a day would be determined by growth, hunger, fussiness clues.

Desiccated liver powder (ugh) could be begun in ever

so small amounts. Kelp powder as a seasoning can be used. Smile as you offer these "goodies."

After nine to ten months add cooked egg yolk, and at a year try to use at least three to six eggs a week. Fowl, fish, lamb, or veal in amounts of one to two tablespoons a day may be added. Softened fruit (banana, apple, pear, avocado) may be mixed with these meats to permit easier ingestion.

Fresh orange, tomato, papaya juice or the pureed fruits are valuable as an alternate fluid. Vitamin C powder can be dissolved in them if the baby suffers from colds or allergies.

At one year the baby is usually getting three or four meals and two or three snacks plus close to a quart of breast or bottle milk a day (enough fluid to urinate well three to five times a day). He gets about two or three ounces of animal, dairy, or plant protein a day, some cereal or whole grain bread and vitamins to match. Brewer's yeast or B complex daily, 250 mg of vitamin C daily, cod liver oil or A and D vitamins and some insurance minerals (kelp or capsule), and some liver product should be given once or twice a week.

At two years of age he is losing his appetite. Those children who fill up on cow's milk may get anemic, so the milk becomes less important, but alternate calcium sources must be adequate. (Aim for close to 1000 mg of calcium per day.) Snacking may work better than three big meals a day.

- *Sample breakfast:* Piece of fruit or juice (plus vitamin C powder), egg or about an ounce of meat or cheese or yogurt plus fruit, 3 to 5 tablespoons of whole grain cereal or bread (plus wheat germ or peanut butter)
- *Snack:* Meat, cheese, fish or milk or vegetable juice drink or carrot cake or oatmeal muffin
- *Lunch:* Soup (pea or bean) plus whole wheat bread and peanut butter
- *Snack:* cottage cheese, fruit, and nut butter

- *Supper:* One ounce of meat, fish, fowl, plus leafy salad, 1 tablespoon of steamed or raw vegetables, a glass of juice or milk
- *Bedtime:* Celery dipped in peanut butter or fruit and yogurt, plus a little dolomite for easier sleep

Dr. Currier's cocktail is for anyone young or old.   One can drink a lot or use it as a snack.   Leave out that which may cause gas or allergy symptoms.

8 ounces milk (raw is best)
1–2 T powdered milk
1–2 eggs
1 T brewer's yeast
1 T wheat germ
1 T lecithin granules
1 T sesame or safflower oil
1 T powdered liver

One might build up to these amounts slowly or use orange, banana, peanut butter, vanilla, etc., to make it more palatable.   Blend.

In between meal snacks should be kept in the bowls about the house to be eaten at any time.   If this destroys the appetite for the next meal, good; it is probably as nourishing as that meal anyway.

Try equal parts of pecans, peanuts, cashews, almonds, raisins, sunflower seeds, pumpkin seeds—all preferably raw and unsalted.

As an alternate raw vegetables cleaned and sliced in a bowl in the refrigerator are convenient.   Old-fashioned peanut butter could be stored next to the vegetables and used as a dip (chilling peanut butter keeps the oil from separating).   Other dips of cottage cheese and avocado or plain yogurt seasoned with onion powder and minced parsley should be near enough to make it all very easy.   Cheese and apple slices together are a good snack.   One-inch chunks of banana rolled in orange juice concentrate and then dipped in wheat germ powder are excellent.

The toughest ones to change are the two- to four-year-olds who have been hooked on the belief that nothing should be eaten unless it tastes sweet or is advertised on television. Ideally, these children should have been programmed in the first year of life so that the only sweet things they know are breast milk and fruit. Because of the big drop in caloric need and appetite at this age, every morsel of food that passes the lips of these children should be highly nutritious. The worst of these kids, the stubborn, irritable, noncompliant preschoolers, present a special problem. Parents think they have no options except maybe passing a feeding tube down the reluctant gullets of these children. Starvation doesn't work; it only makes them more paranoid and hostile. If they would eat better they would feel better, but how to do it?

I suggest the following strategy with these children. (I assume that milk has been stopped for a few weeks and additives screened out and a physical examination and blood test have been made to rule out anemia.) Try substituting honey (it should be pure, raw honey) for sugar. This may be cheating, but one must start somewhere. The idea is to touch everything you want the child to eat with honey. Trap him into eating nutritious foods by utilizing his craving for sweets, then over a period of weeks and months reduce the honey until the child prefers the wholesome taste of good foods. He might even eat liver and onions because he likes the taste of liver and onions.

Many wonder if the frequent eating will lead to obesity. Just the opposite is true. Nibbling (or grazing) seems to be the best way to lose if overweight, or stay the same if just right, or gain if underweight or growing. Nibbling on protein foods and complex carbohydrates (i.e., vegetables) serves to keep the blood sugar from dipping to the range that forces the victim to crave quick sugar.

The refrigerator should be a big salad bowl. Most children prefer vegetables raw—even peas, pea pods, beets (tops and roots), spinach, alfalfa sprouts, onions, peppers, rutabagas, turnips, asparagus, cabbage, broccoli, cauliflower, as well as the traditional lettuce, tomatoes, carrots, radishes and celery.

Then the family sits down to supper. But now because all members have been nibbling all day and everyone's blood sugar is allowing for pleasant social interchange, the usual snarls and elbowing that accompany "feeding time at the zoo" are gone. This last meal should be as simple as possible— really just an excuse to talk over the events of the day.

The raw vegetables can be brought out of the refrigerator, and each can make his own salad. The entree can be bean, pea, or lentil soup, a piece of meat, an omelet or cheese dish. For extra carbohydrate for the rapid growers, whole grain bread or potato or corn would be appropriate. Brown rice is better than white. Try to avoid pasta, canned vegetables, and fruit canned with syrup.

"Dessert" would come two hours later and be fruit best accompanied by nuts, seeds, or cheese. Protein at bedtime allows for easier arising in the morning.

Most recipes for snacks use honey or molasses. These are slightly better than white sugar but should be used only when one is being weaned away from one's sweet tooth. Try to use raisins or dates in recipes calling for sugar. Try to use one fourth of the honey recommended in recipes. Fruits are a natural source to satisfy the sweet craving, but because of their sugar content, they should be eaten with protein to assuage the blood sugar fluctuations.

Cook and puree chicken livers. Season with onion, curry powder, or tarragon. Spread on a stalk of celery. You can call this supper. Some grind up hard-boiled eggs with the liver.

A whole grain cereal (from *Better Living Cookbook*) should stick to the ribs. One cup of the following mix to three cups of water, slowly cooked overnight, serves a lot; store and use frequently.

6 cups whole wheat berries or cracked wheat
6 cups rolled oats
6 cups cornmeal
3 cups brown rice
3 cups buckwheat
3 cups bran
2 cups hulled sunflower seeds.

This diet is fairly high in protein. Most foods except fruit, fats, and refined carbohydrates contain some protein; plant proteins contain similar amounts of protein per calorie. Expensive cuts of meat have too much fat and have no more or better quality protein than legumes.

A six-ounce steak will provide 700 calories and only about 30 grams of usable protein. Two and a half cups of cooked beans will provide the same number of calories and yet deliver 50 percent more usable protein. The latter is low in fat and virtually cholesterol-free.

Peer-group pressure is paramount to the five- to seven-teen-year-old. I have suggested to youngsters in this age group that they nibble on cheese, nuts, seeds, and raw vegetables during school hours. This healthy notion is abandoned as soon as their junk-food addict friends call them "weirdos." Occasionally a teacher can have a tremendous influence for good and make an entire class enthusiastic about good nutrition. In this case, peer pressure works for good. The minority who are still on the marshmallow trip soon conform to the others. Frequently these newly converted "health nuts" become evangelists at home, and the whole family is changed as a result. The Norwegian government provides cheese and fish to each student as a morning snack.

Families with diabetes, alcoholism, obesity, allergies, or stress in the background should be especially careful never to have sugar, ice cream, and white-flour products in their homes. Our findings suggest that children in such families tend to exhibit hyperinsulin response or carbohydrate maladaptation; they get addicted to sweet foods very quickly.

As our children's caretakers we must do what we can to keep them reasoning with a well-nourished neocortex. During the period of transition from the non-nutrients to nutritious foods, you may want to go to the health-food store or co-op for natural foods and vitamins. Some parents buy capsules that contain the B-complex vitamins in powdered form; they pull these apart and shake the contents in minute amounts into peanut butter, soups, and fruits. This is sneaky but effective, since the B-complex vitamins, taken alone, taste like moldy dirt. Build up the amounts given over a period of weeks. The same with dolomite or bone meal—substances that taste like chalk—when milk must be curtailed because of an allergy.

A program of good nutrition has its reward in a calm, cheerful, nonallergic child who, because he feels better, will eat better. A meal should be a fun, social event. Give the hungry house apes and the depressed, surly low-blood-sugar types some raw items or a salad about an hour before mealtime. They should be cheerful and calm when they come to the table, and because they feel better they should be more accepting of the good foods you set before them.

Many peoples and tribes have survived and done well on limited variety. Northern Canadian Indians eat only animals, but they eat the *whole* animal and gnaw on the bones for calcium. Some natives seem to do well on vegetables and fruits but use limestone to get some minerals. For most of us, eating a variety of foods—animal, vegetable, fruit, grains, and dairy products—should allow us to live in a sound body. But because we can no longer trust what comes to us from field and stream, a prudent insurance of vitamins, minerals, and herbs should keep us as healthy as possible, given the not-too-perfect genes we carry.

As a starter, here is a collection of recipes that children like, yet they are full of health-giving ingredients. Note that no sugar is used (some honey to give sweetness), nor chocolate (carob instead), nor white flour (whole wheat, of course). In building your file of family dishes, look for recipes like these that use fresh, unprocessed ingredients, complementary foods, and nutritious substitutes for the commonly used non-nutrients.

Recipes

Fish Casserole

4 pieces (1½–2 lbs.) of any white fish
1 cup fresh mushrooms
1 cup grated jack cheese
2 lbs diced green onion
2 stalks celery, chopped
Chopped parsley
Salt
Pepper
Paprika

Place fish in lightly oiled dish. Lightly salt and pepper. Layer mushrooms, cheese, onion, celery, parsley. Sprinkle with paprika. Bake at 350° for 30 minutes. Serves 4.

Protein Snacks

1 cup peanut butter
½ cup each raisins and
    non-fat dry milk powder
¼ cup sesame seeds
¼ cup honey

Mix together, roll in one-inch balls, refrigerate. Makes about 8 balls.

Granola

  2½ cups raw rolled oats
   1 cup shredded coconut
  ½ cup chopped nuts
  ¼ cup sesame seeds
  ¼ cup raw sunflower seeds
  ½ cup raw wheat germ
  ½ cup honey
  ½ cup oil

Mix and add ½ cup honey and ½ cup oil. Bake at 275° until lightly browned, turning several times. Add dried fruit or raisins after cooking.

Whole Wheat Pizza

  1 cup whole wheat flour
  1 tsp salt
  1 tsp oregano
Pinch of pepper
  2 eggs
  ⅔ cup milk
Corn meal

Beat eggs, add milk, then flour and seasonings. Dust pizza pan with corn meal. Pour in batter, spreading to sides. Arrange topping of your choice. Bake at 425° for 30 minutes. Serves 4.

Natural Candy

  1 cup natural peanut butter
  ¼ cup carob powder
  ¼ cup mashed banana
  2 tsp vanilla

Mix together, shape into balls, and roll in cinnamon. If desired, press a walnut half on top. Store in refrigerator.

Oatmeal Muffins

   2 cups rolled oats, measured
         after grinding in blender
   2 tsp baking powder
   ½ tsp salt
   ¼ cup each oil and honey
   1 egg in a cup—add any fruit
         juice to fill cup
   ½ cup any dried fruit, chopped

Combine oats, baking powder, and salt. Combine honey, oil, juice, egg, and raisins or other fruit. Mix together until blended. Fill and slightly mound greased muffin tins. Bake at 325° for 20 minutes or until done. Makes about 12 muffins.

Quesadillas

Heat corn tortillas on both sides in a little oil. Place slices of jack cheese on one half and roll over. Lettuce, tomatoes, salad greens, chopped green onions may be added.

Spanish Rice

   1 cup brown rice
   2 medium onions, diced
   2 tbs safflower oil
   3 tomatoes, chopped
   2 tbs vinegar
   ½ cup tomato juice
   ½ tsp black pepper
   2 tsp onion powder
   ⅛ tsp garlic powder
   ½ tsp dry, ground horseradish

Sauté onion, green pepper, and rice in oil until rice is dark brown. Add all other ingredients. Simmer 5 minutes. Put in casserole. Bake at 350° for 30 minutes.

Lentils and Rice

    2 large onions
    ¼ cup oil
    1 cup lentils
    4 cups water or stock
    1½ tsp salt
    ¼ tsp white pepper
    ½ cup brown rice

Cut onions into thin slices. Heat oil and fry onions until lightly browned. Set aside half the onions. Rinse lentils and pick over. Put in 3-qt. casserole, add water, bring to boil, and cook covered over low heat for 20 minutes. Add rice, salt, pepper, and the onions with the oil from the frying pan. Continue cooking, covered, over low heat until the lentils and rice are tender but not mushy, about 25 minutes. Top with reserved onions and garnish with parsley. Serves 3 or 4.

Oatmeal Nut Cookies

    3 cups rolled oats
    1 cup whole wheat flour
    1 cup apple juice
    ¼ tsp ground cinnamon
    1 cup raisins
    ½ tsp vanilla
    1 cup warm water
    1 banana mashed
    Dried chopped fruit or
    4 oz. chopped nuts

Mix oats, flour, and apple juice in large bowl until lumps are gone. Stir in cinnamon and raisins. Dissolve vanilla in warm water. Add, mixing thoroughly. Stir in remaining ingredients. Let stand for 15–20 minutes. Mix again and drop by spoonfuls on a nonstick cookie sheet and flatten. Bake 35 minutes at 350°. Cool on rack.

Fudge

1 cup honey
1 cup peanut butter
1 cup carob powder
1 cup unhulled sesame seeds
1 cup sunflower seeds, hulled
½ cup shredded coconut
½ cup chopped dates

Heat honey and peanut butter. Add carob, then remaining ingredients. Pour into oiled 8 x 8 pan and refrigerate to harden. Cut into squares. Each time you make it, cut down on the honey.

Swedish Pancakes

1 cup whole wheat flour
¼ cup honey
1 tsp salt
8 eggs
1 cup milk
¼ cup bran

Mix in blender and drop by tablespoonsful onto hot griddle over a fresh apple slice or piece of precooked bacon. Spread with yogurt or peanut butter—forget the syrup. Makes 16 to 20 "dollar" pancakes.

Tuna Spread or Dip

1 3¼-ounce can tuna
½ cup cream cheese
1 tbs cream
1 cup celery, sliced thin
½ tsp lemon juice
1 tsp onion powder
⅛ tsp black pepper
2 drops tabasco sauce

Put all ingredients except ½ cup sliced celery in blender. Blend until smooth. Mix in small bowl with rest of celery. Cover and chill. Serve as a spread or thin with a little milk for a dip.

Banana-date Cookies

3 bananas
⅓ cup oil
1 cup chopped dates
½ cup chopped walnuts
2 cups rolled oats
1 tsp vanilla
½ tsp salt

Mash bananas. Add dates and oil. Beat with a fork. Add remaining ingredients. Mix lightly. Let stand for oatmeal to absorb moisture. Drop from spoon on ungreased cookie sheet. Bake 25 minutes at 350°. (Watch carefully; they burn easily.) Yield: about 12.

Carob Chip Honey Cookies

1¼ cups whole wheat flour
¾ tsp salt
½ tsp soda
1 tsp vanilla
⅓ cup butter or oil
½ cup honey
1 beaten egg
1 pkg carob chips
1 cup chopped nuts if desired

Sift flour, salt and soda together. Cream shortening and add vanilla, honey, and egg. Add dry ingredients. Mix in carob chips and nuts. Beat well. Drop by teaspoonful on ungreased cookie sheet. Bake at 375° for about 12 minutes. Makes 30–50. Reduce the honey as time goes by.

Bibliography
AND ADDITIONAL HELPS

Books

Airola, Paavo, Ph.D. *Hypoglycemia: A Better Approach.* Phoenix, Ariz.: Health Plus Publishers, 1977.

Feingold, Ben. F., M.D. *Why Your Child Is Hyperactive.* New York: Random House, 1974.

Watson, George, M.D. *Nutrition and Your Mind.* New York: Harper & Row, 1974.

Cleave, T. L., M.R.C.P. *The Saccharine Disease.* New Canaan, Conn.: Keats Publishing Co., 1975.

Smith, Lendon H., M.D. *Improving Your Child's Behavior Chemistry.* Englewood Cliffs, N.J.: Prentice-Hall, 1976.

Baren, Martin, M.D., Robert Liebl, and Lendon Smith, M.D. *Overcoming Learning Disabilities.* Reston, Va.: Reston Publishing Co., Inc., 1978.

Price, Weston, D.D.S. *Nutrition and Physical Degeneration.* Santa Monica, Calif.: Price-Pottenger Foundation, 1970.

Walezak, Michael, M.D. (ed.). *Nutrition—Applied Personally.* La Habra, Calif.: International College of Applied Nutrition, 1975.

Gerrans, Charles, *et al. Encyclopedia of Common Diseases.* Emmaus, Pa.: Rodale Press, 1976.

U.S. Department of Agriculture, *Nutritive Value of Foods*, Bulletin #72. Washington, D.C.: U.S. Government Printing Office, 1977.

Barnes, Broda A., M.D. *Hypothyroidism: The Unsuspected Illness.* New York: Thomas Y. Crowell, 1976.

Williams, Roger. *Physicians' Handbook of Nutritional Science.* Springfield, Ill.: Charles C Thomas, 1975.

Mineral Content of Foods. Hayward, Calif.: Nutrilab, Inc.

Kirschmann, John D. *Nutrition Almanac.* New York: McGraw-Hill, 1975 (paperback).

Brewer, Gail S. *What Every Pregnant Woman Should Know: The Truth about Diet and Drugs in Pregnancy,* New York: Random House, 1977.

Robins, L. *Deviant Children Grow Up.* Baltimore: Williams & Wilkins, 1966.

Help in the Kitchen

Goldbeck, Nikki and David. *The Good Breakfast Book.* Links, a division of Music Sales Corp., 33 W. 60th St., New York, N.Y. 10023, 1976.

Williams, Phyllis. *Nourishing Your Unborn Child.* Nash Publishing Corp., 9255 Sunset Blvd., Los Angeles, Calif. 90069, 1974.

Kende, Margaret and Williams, Phyllis. *The Natural Baby Food Cook Book,* Nash Publishing Corp., 9255 Sunset Blvd., Los Angeles, Calif. 90069, 1972.

School Nutrition Kit. Nutrition Education Center, Inc., P.O. Box 303, Oyster Bay, N.Y. 11771.

Lansky, Vicki. *Feed Me! I'm Yours.* New York: Bantam, 1977.

Seddon, George, and Burrow, Jackie. *Natural Food Book.* Skokie, Ill.: Rand McNally and Co., 1977.

Bailey, Emma. *Better Living Cookbook.* Emmaus, Pa.: Rodale Press, 1977.

Nichols, Virginia. *Cookbook and Guide to Eating,* 3350 Fair Oaks Dr., Xenia, Ohio 45385, 1976.

Berger, Claire. *Claire's Salt Free, Sugar Free, Additive Free, Preservative Free Cookery.* P.O. Box 1401, Englewood, Colo. 80150.

Sloan, Sara. *A Guide for Nutra Lunches and Natural Foods.* SOS Printing Co., Inc., Atlanta, Ga., 1977.

Newsletters

Linus Pauling Institute of Science and Medicine, 2700 Sam Hill Road, Menlo Park, Calif. 94025.

Developmental Disabilities Prevention Center, Inc., P.O. Box 1282, Medford, Ore. 97501.

The Institute for Child Behavior Research, 4758 Edgeware Road, San Diego, Calif. 92116.

New Jersey Hypoglycemia Association, Box 192, Ridgewood, N.J. 07451.

International Childbirth Education Association, Inc., Box 5852, Milwaukee, Wis. 53220.

La Leche League International, 9616 Minneapolis Ave., Franklin Park, Ill. 60131.

Association for Children with Learning Disabilities, 5225 Grace St., Pittsburgh, Pa. 15326.

Missouri Association for Hyperactive Children, Inc., Box 452, Jefferson City, Mo. 65101.

Doctors, Dentists

International Academy of Preventive Medicine, 10409 Town and Country Way, Houston, Tex. 77024.

Orthomolecular Medical Society, 2340 Parker St., Berkeley, Calif. 94704.

Huxley Institute, 1114 First Ave., New York, N.Y. 10021.

Index